Goddess Star Monroe

Pole Essentials

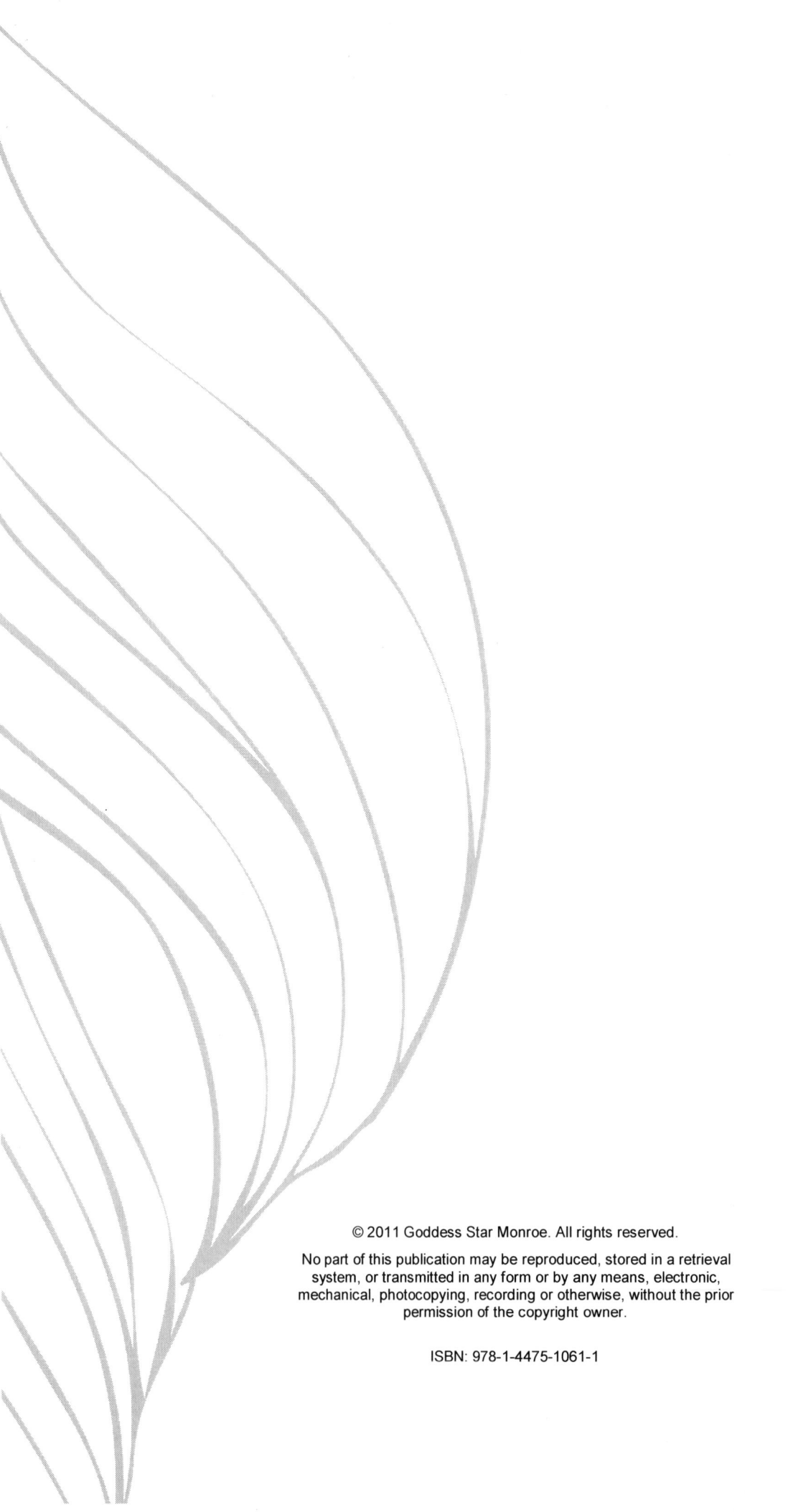

© 2011 Goddess Star Monroe. All rights reserved.

No part of this publication may be reproduced, stored in a retrieval system, or transmitted in any form or by any means, electronic, mechanical, photocopying, recording or otherwise, without the prior permission of the copyright owner.

ISBN: 978-1-4475-1061-1

Contents

Foreword from Zoraya Judd 4

Expressing my gratitude 5

Why Pole Dancing? 6

How to use this book 7

Essential Tricks and Tips 8

Body Essentials for Pole Dancing 9

Just for fun – What's your secret pole personality? 10

Meet the rest of the team 13

Level One 15

Level Two 36

Level Two 37

Level Three 55

Level Four 69

Goddess Star Monroe's Expertise and Qualifications 90

What other Pole Instructors say about Pole Dancing 92

Juicy Resources 96

It goes deeper 98

A note from me to you 99

Important.

The information in this book reflects the author's experiences and opinions and is not intended to replace medical advice.

Before beginning this or any nutritional or exercise programme, please consult your doctor to be sure it is appropriate.

Foreword from Zoraya Judd

My name is Zoraya Judd and I have been pole training for a little over 3 years now. I started after the birth of my second son when a dear friend invited me to a pole fitness class. When I got there I was so amazed at the power and control that the students had in order to hold their body out and flip up the pole. I was instantly hooked.

After 6 months, I took over the class and started teaching it. I was so passionate and driven. I had found something that was so empowering and beautiful. Without being sexual, I felt so sexy and in control. Pole changed my life and my body in ways I would have never imagined possible.

Two weeks after that, I was entered into my first ever pole competition. I had ZERO dance background and no gymnastics training and I had never even tried to do a bunch of pole combos for any amount of time in a row. The competition required a 3-5 minute routine so because I was so uncomfortable with floor work or any kind of dance, I created a 3+ minute routine only on the pole. Those two weeks were the first time I had ever trained more than twice a week. I trained so hard I had lost most of the skin behind both my knees. The anxiety and nerves I got were indescribable and almost addictive. I created an alter ego to step out of my head for the performance. Man, did it help! I won first place in the advanced division in the first ever Utah Pole competition.

My first competition created a monster in me. The adrenaline I got from it was indescribable. Shortly after I entered into my second competition, I received my pro card. My 5th competition was in Zurich, Switzerland where I became one of the top 10 pole dancers in the world. Immediately afterwards, I went to Tokyo to compete for the International title and I won the title "Pole Art Champion 2011".

I love spreading the love of pole through example, performances, competitions, workshops and private instruction. I have met the most amazing people and have the most amazing sponsors and supporters. My fans make this journey breathtaking and I thank them for believing in me.

I initially met Star in 2010 when I hosted a workshop in the UK but got to spend more time with her in 2011 when she flew over from the UK to stay with my family in Utah. We had 3 days to train 10 hours on the pole, 6 hours at the gym and 2 hours of flexibility. For me, this is life, an everyday intense lifestyle - I sleep, breathe, eat and live for perfecting my goals. I was so excited that Star flew thousands of miles to experience the life of the Judds.

Each day Star was with me, she ate what I ate, trained how I train and pushed pole to the limit. No matter how hard I pushed Star, she never gave up. In those 3 days I am pretty sure I experienced every side of Star but she never caved. I am so proud of her. She is SO driven and such a hard worker. She conquered our training and then some. She took notes, asked questions, reviewed, and studied. Star is definitely an amazing inspirational role model. She knows what it takes to achieve goals. I wish we were closer to each other.

If you want something bad enough, it takes work. But everything you work REALLY hard for is usually the most rewarding. Thank you Star for flying all that way. Thank you for believing I was the one that could help you grow. Thank you for not punching me in the face for pushing you so hard. You are such an amazing individual and I am so proud to call you a dear friend. Keep sharing the love of pole and encouraging those to grow. You are an amazing woman.

My advice to you all is to find something you are passionate about and CONQUER IT. You CAN have it all. It won't be easy, but it is ALL worth it. I want to thank you guys for taking the time to read this, for your support and for the drive you all give me.

http://www.zorayajudd.com/

http://www.ZenArtsLa.com/

Expressing my gratitude

A big massive, gorgeously, sparkly thank you to Sarah London, my assistant instructor who painstakingly applied all my amendments without a murmur of complaint.

Goddess sparkles to Sj, Sarah, Julia, Claire and Karen for being exceptional pole models. I am very proud and honoured that you are all part of my life.

To the fantastic Ian J for taking all the photos (I don't think he minded!).

To all my pole assistants that have helped me run the most fabulously, exciting classes throughout these past 10 years. A special mention to Hege Bergum - I just adore you darling girl xxx

Special gratitude to Ami Wood whose patience and diligence to detail enabled this book to be as wonderful as it is.

And finally....

To my son, George Gibbons who I love with all my heart. You make me laugh, smile, cry and shout (sometimes all at the same time!) and very, very, very proud to be called your mum. There is no one like you George, you are amazing! Xxx

Why Pole Dancing?

Pole dancing is all about women, our curves, our sensuality and our femininity. Women are known for their determination and persistence and this is where you will have the chance to fully explore all these qualities.

Pole dancing is a beautiful and elegant skill that when mastered and practised, will make you look and feel amazing. Your body will change, becoming more toned and supple, your legs will look like you've been a dancer for years, body image and confidence 'va va vooms', and wow, will you have some party tricks to show your friends!

I still remember the first time I tried pole dancing. I dragged my friend Jo up to London to a top gentlemen's club where we had far too many glasses of wine, cavorted, and played around on the neon stage pretending like we knew it all. That was over 10 years ago - I was hooked then and still am now.

I have watched the pole dancing / fitness industry grow from teaching small groups of girls easy pole tricks in strip clubs to the amazing strong and athletic skill it is today. With pole dancing schools opening up across the globe this is one fitness trend that is here to stay.

Personally, I love how pole dancing has transformed my body. From always being bottom heavy with weak arms, at 40 years old my body has never looked so good. I have defined arms, strong abdominals, my body is beautifully balanced and I can do tricks on the pole anybody half my age would be in awe of.

Pole dancing gives you strength, power and agility. It ultimately puts you in control of your body. I always tell my students that we only ever get one body in this lifetime and it is our responsibility to look after it and be the best we can be. Well, pole dancing gives you that fabulous, fun opportunity AND you get to wear high heels whilst doing it too!

It is always an honour and a privilege to watch my students grow from shy, body image conscious girls to strong, independent women. Pole dancing opens the door to our sensuality and femininity - both true essences to a strong, happy and secure woman.

So come on in gorgeous one, see how the wonderful word of pole dancing can help you blossom and grow into the true woman you were born to be.

How to use this book

I have devised my 'Pole Essentials' to be just that - an 'essential' addition to your pole training and dancing. Use it as a reference manual, a pole journal or just as an inspiring reminder that you can achieve anything you desire.

There is information on who I am, my essential tricks, tips, and body fundamentals, which are vital to your pole practice.

Just for fun (because pole dancing is fun!), there is a quiz for you to discover your inner pole personality and then I have designed levels 1 - 4 for you to learn, progress, make notes and be inspired from.

At the back, there is information on my qualifications and expertise, stories from other top pole dancers, a juicy resource section and a special, sparkly note from me to you.

All the pole dancers in this book are my students and started with no experience at all. With dedication, practice and patience you too can achieve everything in this book.

The levels are graded on difficulty and experience. Level 1 is the foundation to a strong pole practice and is essential to all new pole dancers. If you are new to pole dancing, please start here. Level 2 is equivalent to a basic intermediate practice and levels 3 and 4 are full of intermediate to advanced moves that require deeper strength, control and balance.

If you are new to any level, then please start at the beginning and work your way through the moves. I have designed each level so that you progressively build your strength and skills by following the set order in which the moves are laid out.

If you are an experienced pole dancer using this book, then feel free to dip in and out of any level for tricks, tips, reminders and inspiration.

You will see I have included all the basic instructions for each move and added my own notes to help you with your practice. There is also space for you to scribble, doodle and make your own notes - essential, I feel, when learning a new skill.

As pole dancing is an ever-evolving method, there are SO many different names for each move. I have tried my best to keep the names as generic as possible but have at times used the names that I christened the moves when I was learning. Feel free to scribble out and pen the name of your choice.

Just a note on your dominant arm and less dominant arm:
I am right handed so my dominant arm is right, less dominant arm is left.

Essential Tricks and Tips

I want you to be the best you can on the pole so please take your time to read my essential tricks and tips before you delve deeply into the levels.

1. Please make sure you warm your body up before any pole practice. Do something that raises your body temperature such as dancing and body weight exercises i.e. squats and lunges. Add in mobility work for your shoulders, wrists and hips too.

2. Have a plan when practising your moves. The formula I follow is this:
   - 3 - 10 repetitions of each of the basic strength exercises on the pole (on both sides)
   - 5 - 10 mins of spins and transitions
   - Practise climbing variations and sitting on the pole
   - Inverting and aerial work
   - Stretch and be proud!

3. Over a period of time as you become more familiar with the moves, you can start combining the moves to design your own routine.

4. Take regular breaks and drinks lots of water.

5. Grab your girlfriend to practise with. Great for motivation and you can spot each other on the more challenging moves.

6. Ideal clothing is a pair of shorts / hot pants, a vest top and sports bra. You need bare arms and legs for most of the moves - especially as you progress through the levels with more skin needed as you move into Levels 3 and 4.

7. Make sure your skin has no body lotion or oil on it. This prevents slipping.

8. Understand that you may accumulate a few bruises when starting out and trying new moves. As you gain more strength and control, bruises will disappear. I recommend arnica tablets and cream if your skin bruises like a peach.

9. When starting your pole practice I recommend bare feet to ALL my students. As you become more skilled in the levels, shoes are an option for you to dance in.

   When learning anything new ALWAYS practise in bare feet.

   When putting routines together and moving through transitions I LOVE to play in my shoes - it makes me feel sexy, womanly and my posture feels great. See the resources at the back for more information on shoes.

10. Grip is always an issue with students, whether new or experienced. I recommend liquid chalk, or 'Dry Hands' for your hands and rubbing alcohol or window cleaner to clean the pole. Have a towel handy to wipe the pole. See the resources at the back for more details.

11. Always complete your pole workout with a full body stretch. If you want to increase your flexibility then a more structured flexibility routine needs to be sourced and followed.

Body Essentials for Pole Dancing

It's all about posture, posture, posture gorgeous one. Here are my body essentials that will help you look sensational on and off the pole.

1. When standing next to the pole, stand tall and elongate your spine. Imagine you are growing taller from the inside out. This is pretty easy to do but more challenging when moving in and out of your moves on the pole. Practise, practise, practise.

2. Pole dancing is great for your core. Did you know that your core is NOT just your abdominals? Your core runs from your pelvic floor (between your legs) to the top of your neck. The main muscles you need to be aware of are your abdominals (there are four layers!), your pelvic floor and your back and shoulder muscles.

3. Essential cues to make you stronger and more elegant on and off the pole are:

    - Shoulders down and back - this basically means keep your shoulders away from your ears when you spin, transition and pull up on the pole.

    - Keep your abdominals drawn in - think about pulling your belly button towards your spine.

    - Breathe! - I know, I know this sounds simple but most of my students will hold their breath when trying something new, which just makes it even more challenging.

4. When walking around the pole without shoes on - walk on your tiptoes. It makes it easier for you to transition in and out of moves and gives you a great workout for you legs too! Keep your head up, eyes forward, smile and be proud. Release your inner GODDESS!

5. When moving into any spin, resist the urge to 'Jump" into the spin, focus on drawing your shoulders down and back, lifting up and floating effortlessly into each spin. Trust me, with practice this does get easier.

6. Listen to yourself when pole dancing, if you can hear your footsteps on the floor when you land or you make a "thudding " sound when you move in and out of moves on the pole - you are not using your upper body or core strength. Think light, think ballet dancer or ninja. Softly, elegantly, quietly is the way to go.

7. All moves in this book were performed on a static pole but can be performed on a spinning pole too.

Just for fun – What's your secret pole personality?

We all have a secret side to us that is waiting to be unleashed. Answer the following questions, add up your answers and discover your ultimate pole personality!

It's the weekend and it's all yours - what do you do?

a. Do something energetic - have a pole jam, go sprint training or sign up for a martial arts class
b. I am deciding how many parties I can attend in one night - is nine too many?
c. Download some awesome music and dance the weekend away
d. Go for a walk, bake a cake, enjoy some well earned "me" time
e. I am polishing up my rubber catsuit for the Fetish Ball this evening

If your house were on fire, what would you save?

a. Saving anything? I'll be putting the fire out!
b. I'll be frantically saving my wardrobe
c. My well-worn ballet shoes
d. The family photos
e. My rare jewelled whip collection

What do you love about yourself?

a. My wisdom
b. My many admirers
c. That I can do the splits
d. My baking skills
e. My cleavage

Your dream holiday?

a. An intense boot camp in the middle of the jungle
b. A stunning private villa with all mod cons just outside Ibiza Old Town
c. Salsa with the locals in Cuba
d. Taking deep cleansing breaths in the mountains in France
e. Gleaning make up tips from the lady-boys in Bangkok

How do you feel about being a woman?

a. Being a woman is brilliant - you have all this power
b. Woman? I prefer being a girl - thank you!
c. I barely notice it
d. I am a natural nurturer and carer. I use my intuition wisely
e. I'm goddamn sexy!

Where are you in your element?

a. In the gym
b. Harvey Nichols in London
c. The dance floor
d. Outside or in my kitchen - cooking up a storm
e. In my S&M dungeon

What is your fashion sense?

a. I have my own style and I know how to rock it
b. Anything expensive and sparkly
c. Lycra
d. Classic and comfortable
e. Tight and figure hugging

Describe the animal in you...

a. Leopard
b. Kitten
c. Gazelle
d. Lioness
e. Black widow spider

Now gorgeous one, tally up your score and all is revealed on the next page...

Mostly a

WARRIOR WOMAN

You are one strong and determined woman. You know what you want and how to go about getting it. You are grounded, fierce and assertive. You don't back down from a challenge.

Mostly b

SEX KITTEN

Goodness me, you are all sweetness and light! A Princess of course! You love to be adored and you are normally surrounded by many admirers, all wanting to spoil you rotten.

Mostly c

DANCER

You love to move and enjoy your body. When the music plays, you just can't keep still. You are always the first one on the dance floor.

Mostly d

EARTH GODDESS

Practical, no nonsense and caring. You are strong and loving. Everyone loves to be around you. Your house is always full of children, friends and family.

Mostly e

VIXEN

The dark, mysterious one. You are alluring, sensual but can be deep and moody at times too. You are always up to something mischievous. It has to be a special man to handle you!

Meet the rest of the team

SJ

SJ has been pole dancing for over 3 years; she is a dance student and is British Sign Language Level 2 qualified. Her big dream is to teach the deaf how to dance. She loves the overall fitness she achieves from pole dancing and saysit's great for meeting lovely friends. SJ is strutting her stuff on page 16.

Sarah

Sarah has been pole dancing for over 3 years and works as my wonderful assistant instructor. She has a solid dance background and is a fabulous burlesque teacher and performer. Sarah is currently learning more about Pilates so she can build her own Pilates client base. Sarah is super flexible and loves how strong her body feels from pole dancing. Discover Sarah on page 18.

Julia

Julia has been pole dancing for just over 3 years and loves how pole has helped her confidence and self-esteem. Julia is a regular performer at my evening events and is talented and oh so slightly naughty. She has just finished studying for a degree in business studies and is about to launch her own events company. Julia pops up in Level 2, page 38.

Claire

Claire has been pole dancing for 4 years and is a regular in my advanced classes. By day, she works as a pharmacist and is a proud mum to three children. She loves to shock people by telling them that her hobby is pole dancing. Claire is also a regular performer for my evening events and always wows the audience with her skills on the pole. Find Claire on the pole, page 41.

Karen

Karen has been pole dancing with myself for over 6 years now. She has seen me through many ups and downs yet she has been so faithful and trusting in my pole teachings. She is my pole buddy, and I regularly practise with Karen on Saturday mornings. Outside pole, Karen is an events organiser. Karen is showing you her skills on page 59.

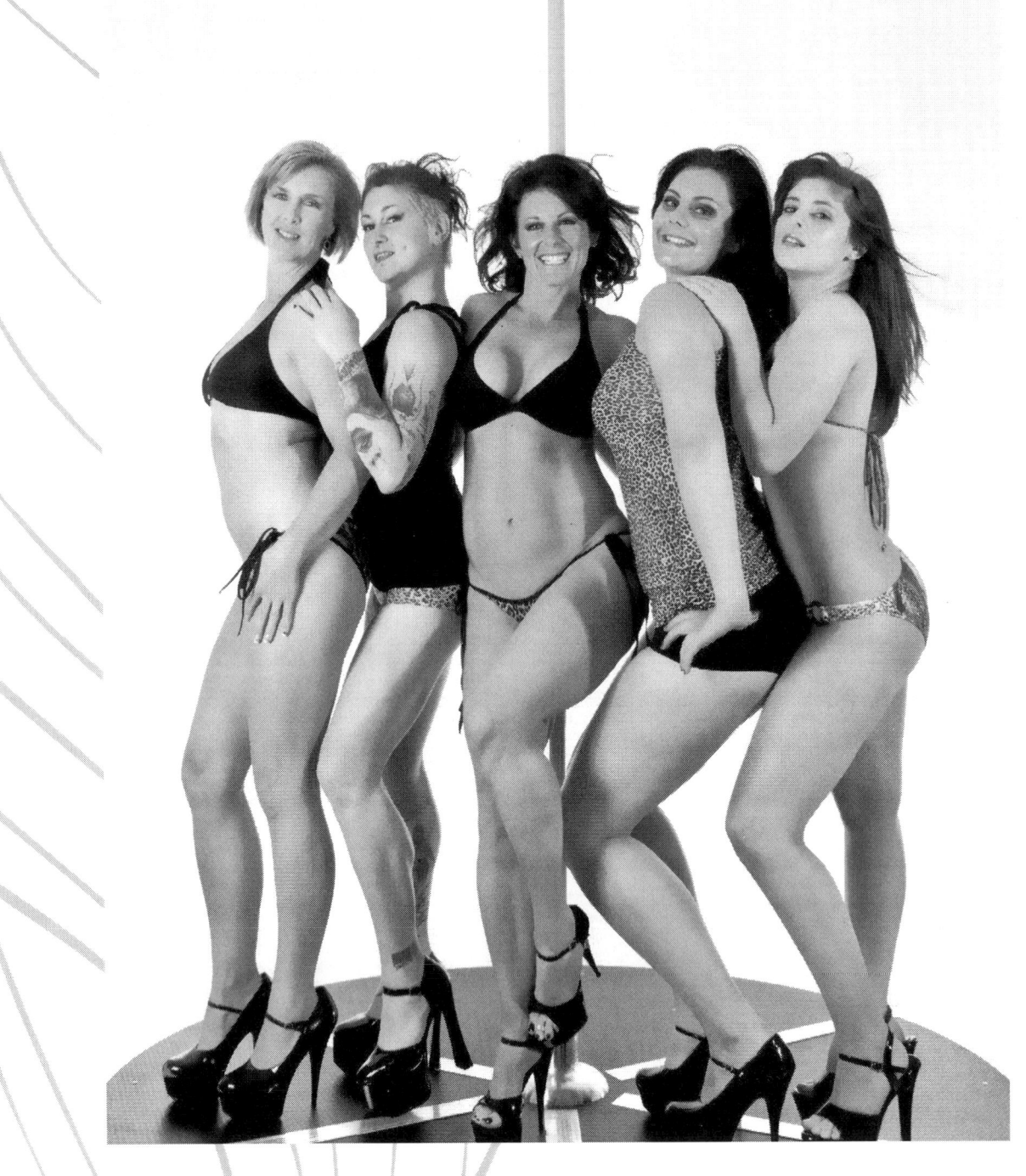

Happy to be pole dancing!

Level One

Level one is designed for the woman completely new to the world of pole dancing. In this level, you will find the most comprehensive set of foundational pole skills that are at the very essence of your wonderfully strong and sensual pole-dancing alter ego.

Level one is all about progressively increasing your pole repertoire, building up and rocking out your strength and coordination on the pole. There is always a massive learning curve at this level and you will be introduced to pole specific strength training, spins, transitions and climbs.

Take your time and enjoy the ride. What you learn here will serve you beautifully as you gently progress through the levels.

Level 1

The Pole Walk

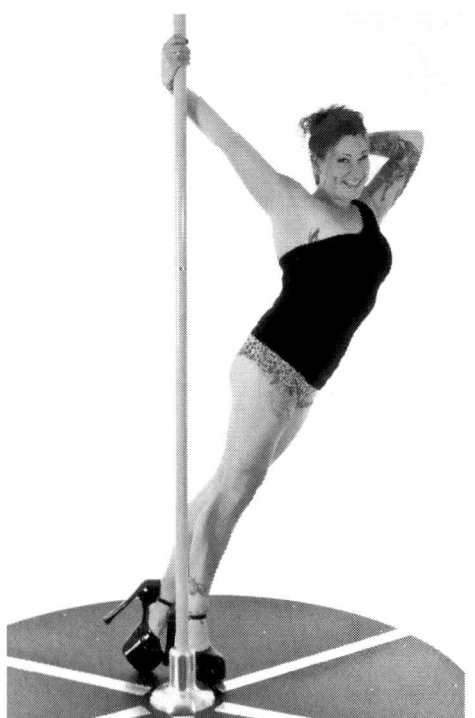

- Weight is on the balls of your feet
- Feet stay close to the bottom of the pole
- Shoulders down and back, chest lifted
- Dominant arm high on pole
- Less dominant arm on hip or behind head
- Lean body out from pole as you walk around
- Step and drag the other foot forward
- Continue around the pole
- Repeat in the other direction

GSM's notes

"Have fun with this one, I always imagine I am slightly lazy or a little tipsy. It slows me down and stops me getting dizzy!"

Your notes:

_____
_____
_____
_____

Level One

Lazy Stripper

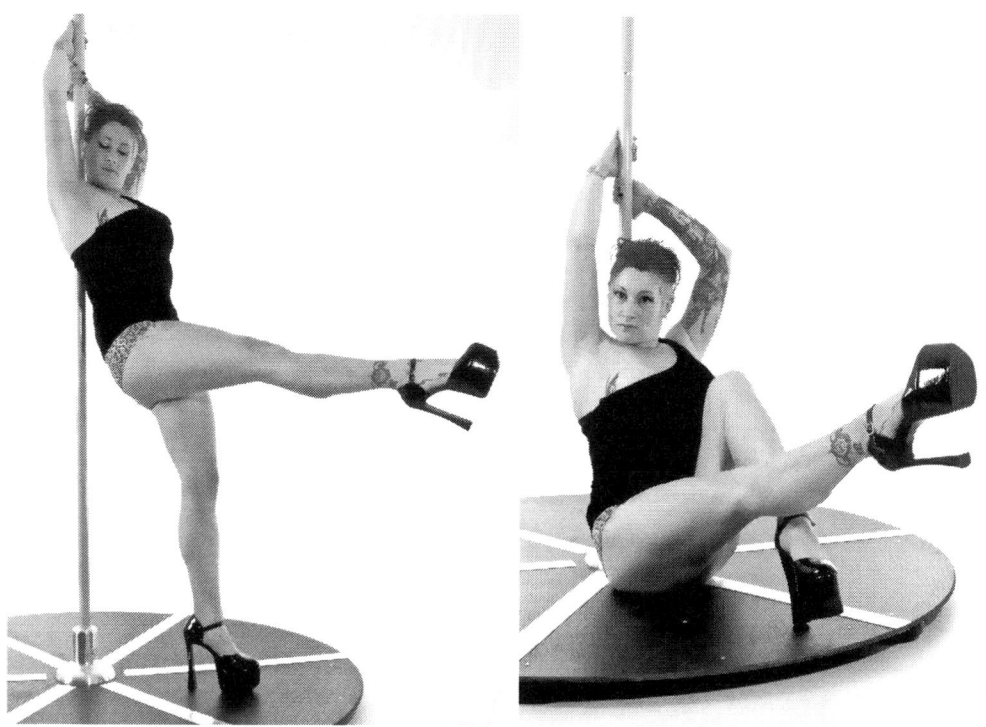

- Back to pole, resting sacrum (base of spine) against pole, hands hold the pole above head
- Step out with one foot, and place your weight on this foot
- Other leg lifts and extends, foot is pointed
- Loosen grip on hands and slide down to floor onto bottom
- Come onto your knees and stand up

GSM's notes

"This is a great transition move and pretty simple to do. Just make sure you step out far enough, otherwise you will land on your foot!"

Your notes:
___
___
___
___

Level One
360° Dip around the Pole

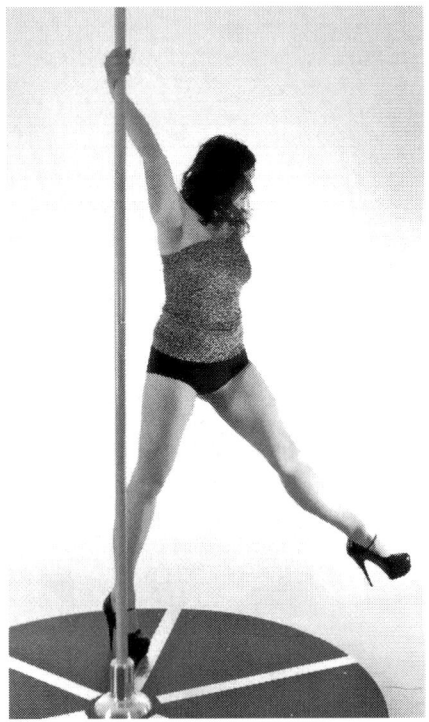

- Stand feet together facing the pole
- Dominant arm high on the pole, you can put the other hand on too if you feel more secure
- Weight is on the dominant leg
- Sweep the other leg around in a big circle 360° to join the other foot - you will be pivoting and lifting off the dominant leg
- You can add an optional pivot turn to complete this move - turn inwards towards the pole
- Repeat the other way

GSM's notes

"Love this move. This baby is always in my routines as I can flow in and out of it effortlessly. Remember to keep a great upright posture and your shoulders down and back."

Your notes:

_____
_____
_____
_____

Level One
Pole Park

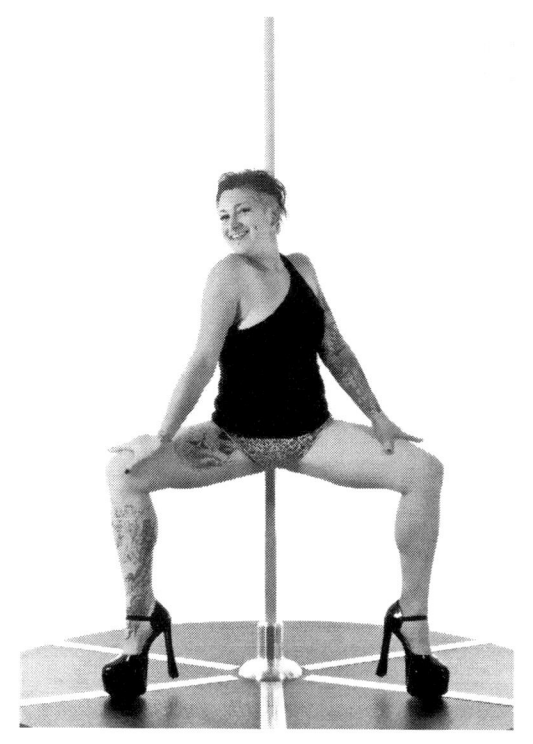

GSM's notes

"Adding a bit of sassy attitude to your pole practice and a great workout for those legs! You can add a 360° Dip around the Pole so it goes Dip - Turn - Park!"

Your notes:
___
___
___
___

Level One
Front Hook

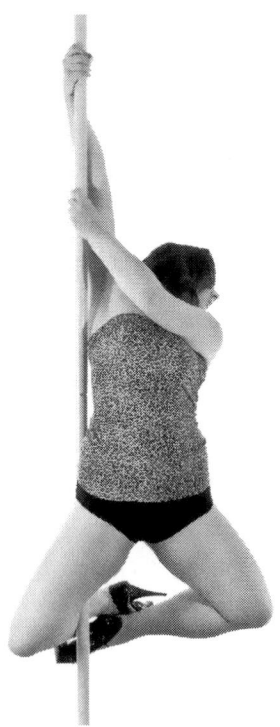

- Stand side on to pole with your dominant arm next to the pole
- Both hands on pole, dominant hand high, less dominant hand at chest height
- Lift inside leg up first and hook onto pole, so it sits in the back of your knee
- Pull up with arms as you lift your outside leg up and spin
- Try to bring heels together
- Lead with chest
- Step down and finish
- Repeat other side

GSM's notes

"A pretty little spin with a couple of exit options. You can step out of it but you could also land delicately on your knees and move into floor work."

Your notes:
_____
_____
_____
_____

Level One
Back Hook

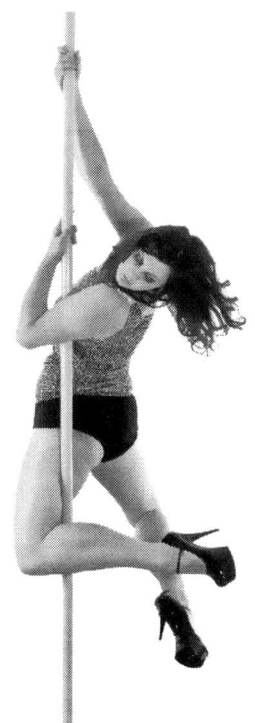

- Stand side on to pole with your dominant arm on the outside
- You are now going to be spinning backwards
- Dominant arm high, less dominant arm chest height, hug pole with this inside arm
- Outside leg sweeps backwards as you pull up with your arms
- Lift inside leg and bring feet towards each other
- Land gently with knees on the floor
- Repeat other side

GSM's notes

"This is just the same as the Front Hook but you are now spinning backwards. I love this move and as you become more confident you can link this move with lots of other spins and inverts."

Your notes:
___
___
___
___

Level One

Basic Spin

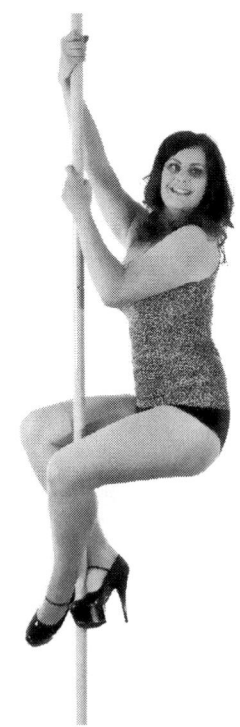

- Start standing side on to the pole
- Dominant arm high, less dominant arm shoulder height
- Weight on inside foot
- Use arms to pull your weight up as you sweep your outside leg round - back of ankle contacts the pole in front
- Inside foot lifts off floor and sits against the back of the pole
- Repeat other way

GSM's notes

"Imagine the legs are in a curtsy position. If my girls get confused I ask them to stand in the same position with their feet on the floor around the pole. Doing a spin and coordinating the feet at the same time can confuse most of us - don't worry, it will all fall into place."

Your notes:

_____
_____
_____
_____

Level One
Double Knee Spin

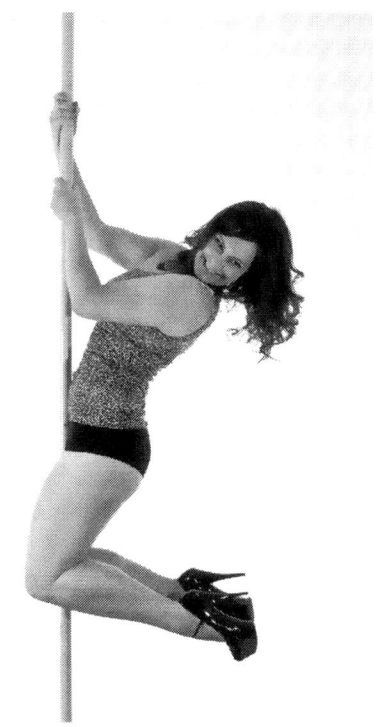

- Start facing the pole - hands are high on the pole - dominant arm is high
- Shoulders down and back
- Weight on the dominant leg and sweep the less dominant leg around
- Pull up with your arms, whilst keeping shoulders down
- Both knees to pole - make sure it is your inside knees contacting the pole and pull your belly to the pole
- Spin down gently to your knees
- To help, you can focus your eyes onto the pole where your knees are going to go
- Repeat on the other side

GSM's notes

"A pretty safe and secure spin when you place the pole correctly. A lot of my girls let the pole feed right up to the top of their inner thighs and then wonder why they get stuck. The trick is to place the pole between your knees."

Your notes:

_____
_____
_____
_____

Level One
Goddess Sit

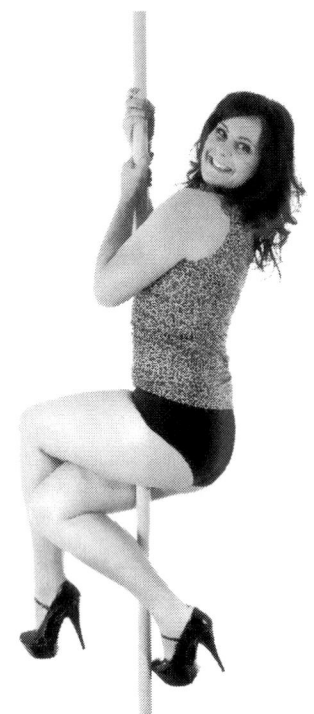

- First, determine which leg crosses over which when you sit - you will mimic this on the pole
- Step your feet forward of the pole so your pubic bone is next to the pole, knees bent
- Both hands head height, dominant arm is top
- Shoulders down, pull your body weight up, take legs forward of pole
- Knees still bent
- Cross your top leg over the bottom one
- You can hook the bottom foot around the pole and when secure you can let go with your hands - make sure you stay upright towards the pole

GSM's notes

"This move should come with an ouch factor rating of 10 / 10. Be prepared! When starting this move it will feel like a Chinese burn against your inner thighs. Trust me, it gets better!"

Your notes:
___
___
___
___

Level One

Climbing

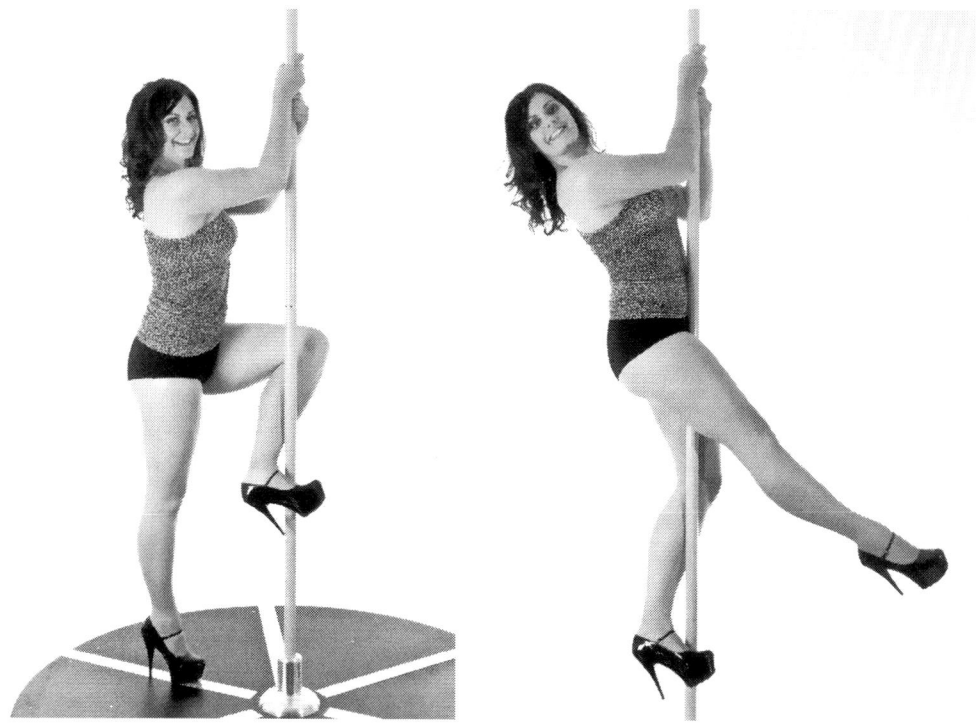

- Hands high on pole, dominant arm high
- Stronger leg on the pole - foot on the inside, knee on the outside, leg is high on the pole (imagine a box underneath you that you are stepping up from)
- Pull yourself up the pole using your arms and tummy muscles
- Imagine there is a magnet on your pubic bone and pull your body up flush to the pole
- Extend the trailing leg forwards and grip with your inner thighs
- Keep your bottom foot flexed as it will help to keep you secure
- Option - you can move into the Goddess Sit (page 24).

GSM's notes

"I remember when I first started pole dancing and wow, this move was so hard. This is where you need your upper body strength. Keep practising and it will come."

Your notes:

_____
_____
_____
_____

Level One
Peekaboo Pose

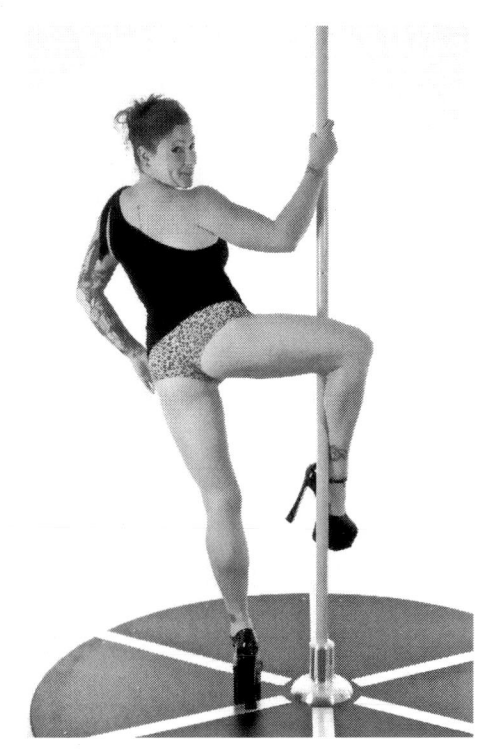

GSM's notes

"A cheeky little pose, ideal to show off your bottom and legs to your lucky audience! It gives you a rest from the pole spins and strength work. You can add this on to the end of your Basic Spin."

Your notes:
_____
_____
_____
_____

Level One
Cheeky Pose

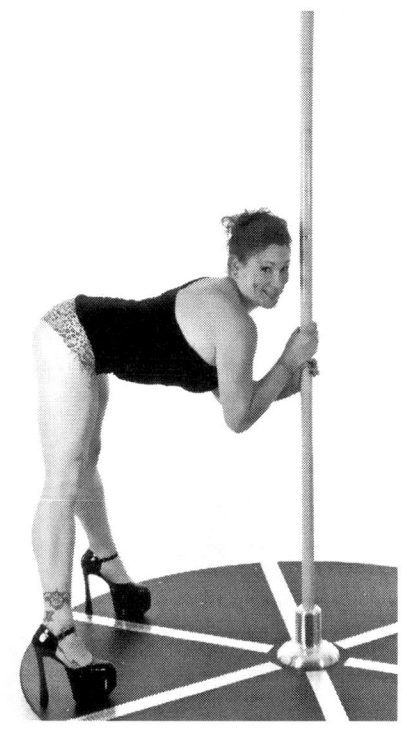

GSM's notes

"The trick here is to keep your back flat and lift your bottom up as you glide the hands down the pole. You can do this with your feet together or apart depending on your mood. Walk hands slowly back up the pole to stand."

Your notes:
_____
_____
_____
_____

Level One
Sexy Crouch

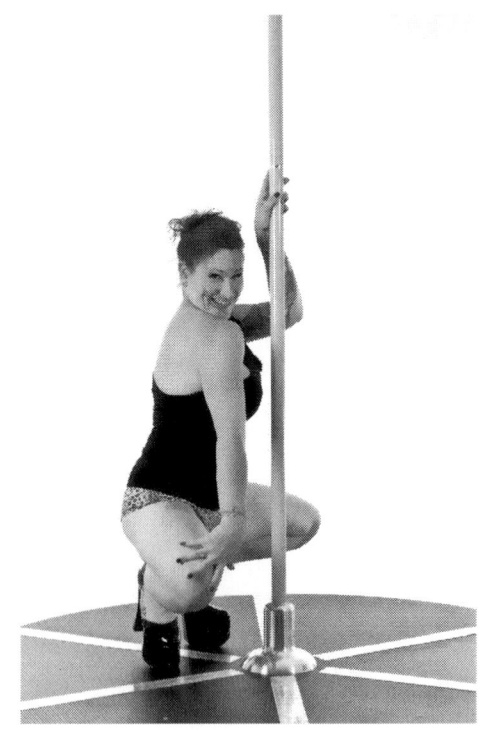

GSM's notes

"Gorgeous one! It's all about the flow. These poses give you time to breathe and chill before you start spinning, climbing, and inverting again. Always accentuate your curves as you move in and out of this move — lead up and out with your bottom first and then your boobs in a snaking action."

Your notes:

_____
_____
_____
_____

Level One
Body Roll

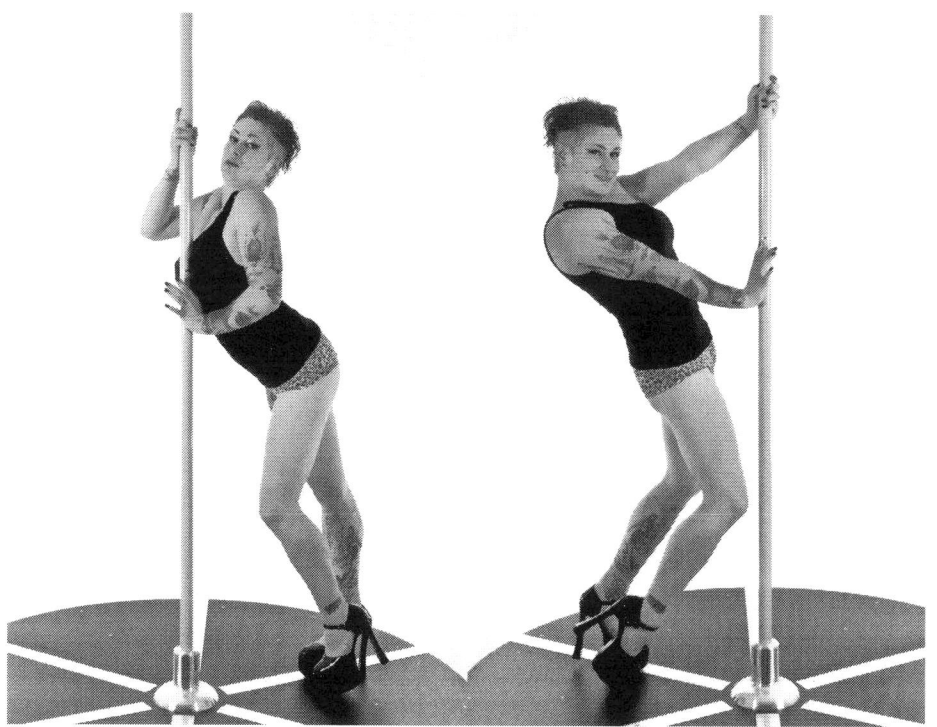

- Start with weight on the balls of your feet facing the pole
- Dominant arm high, less dominant arm low
- Lean chest into pole, followed by hips
- Then lean body away from pole leading from your back, then your hips
- You are looking for a 'snake like' undulation with your body

GSM's notes

"Trust me with this, unless you have some dance experience this one will need some practice. Try it in front of a mirror leaning on a door frame - you can have a giggle whilst learning!"

Your notes:

_____
_____
_____
_____

Level One
Maiden Pose

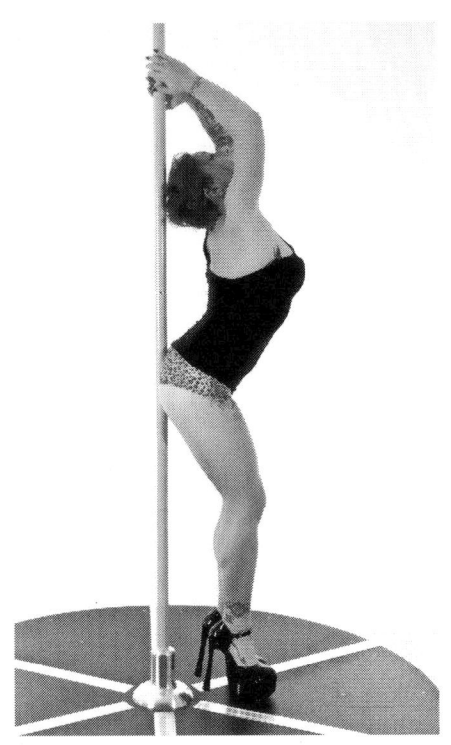

GSM's notes

"*This is a super sexy move guaranteed to show off all your womanly curves! Use it in the middle of a routine and just 'pause' in it for maximum effect!*"

Your notes:
_____
_____
_____
_____

Level One
Back Arch

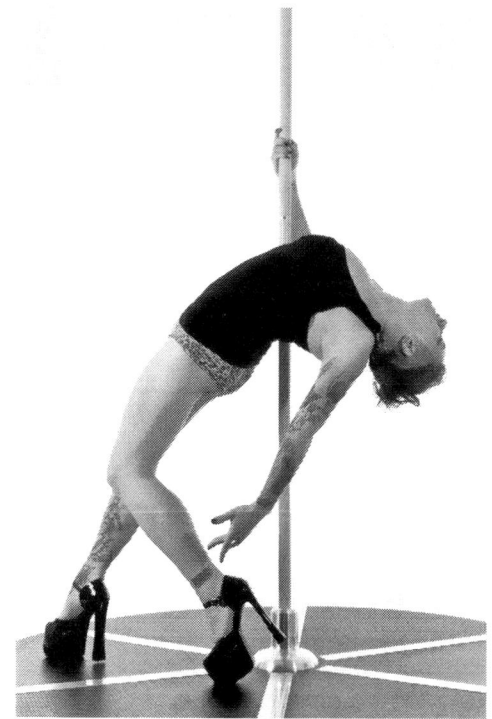

- Start standing side on to pole
- Dominant arm is high on pole
- Step both feet forwards - they are slightly apart
- Weight on your inside leg
- Arch through your upper back
- Slide down leading with your head
- You will lay leading head, shoulders, back, bottom onto the floor
- You can add this move on to a Front Hook

GSM's notes

"Sometimes my hand gets stuck, sometimes I just slide right down without any grip and sometimes it works perfectly. Make sure the feet are far enough out, otherwise you will land on them - ouch!"

Your notes:
_____
_____
_____
_____

Level One
Hair Flick

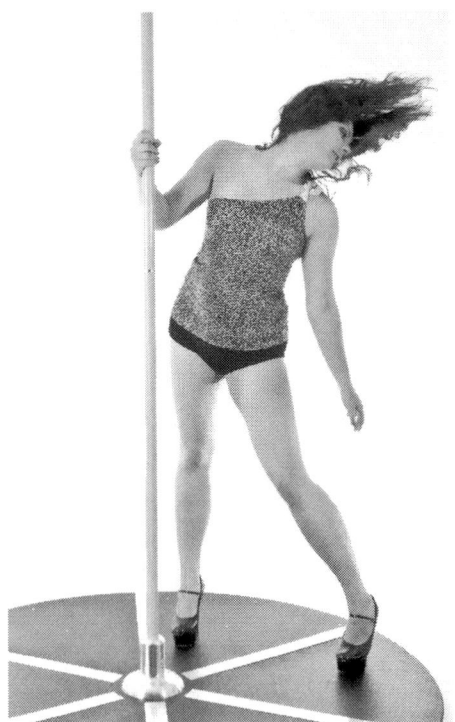

- You can do this standing or whilst spinning to give your move a little more va va voom!
- Drop your outside ear to your shoulder and sweep your head to the other side in a quick, clean motion

GSM's notes

"I always wonder how I look when I do this but hey, it feels so good I just don't care! Any neck issues - steer away."

Your notes:
___
___
___
___

Level One

Tuck to the Sides

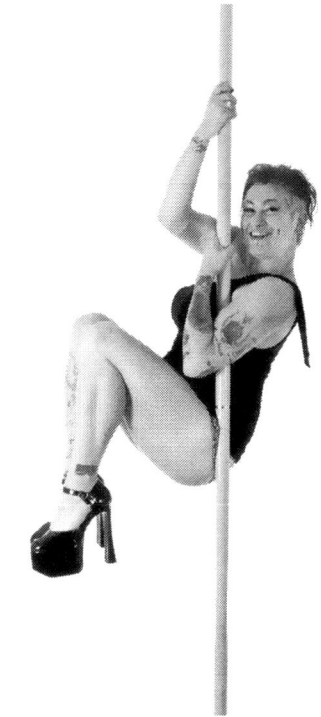

- Body to side of the pole
- Less dominant arm hugs the pole chest height
- Dominant arm high
- Body is slightly in front of pole
- Shoulders down and back
- Pull up, raise knees to tummy and hold
- Repeat both sides
- This is a great conditioning move!

GSM's notes

"You've gotta love the Tuck! I make all my girls do these at the start of every session, whatever their level. Super great for toning up your arms and tummy and they build up your strength for future moves."

Your notes:

_____
_____
_____
_____

Level One
Half Bracket Hold

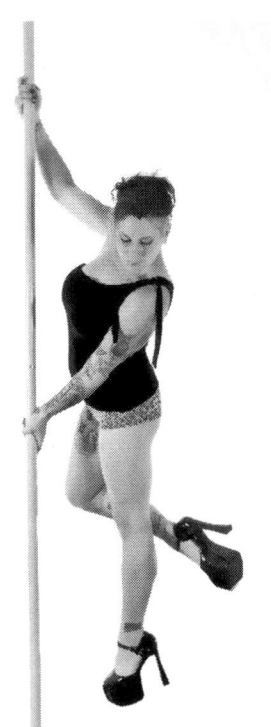

- Start on tiptoes facing the pole
- Dominant arm high, less dominant arm low (fingers facing down)
- Rotate shoulders down and back
- Pull up with top arm and push with bottom to lift feet off the floor, hold!
- Lower with control
- Repeat other side

GSM's notes

"Ooooo, get ready gorgeous ones, this is a super, duper strengthening move. When you nail this move, you know you are getting stronger! Have patience as this is a tough move, even if you can just pull yourself up a teeny tiny bit – BE PROUD!"

Your notes:

_____
_____
_____
_____

Level One
Windmill

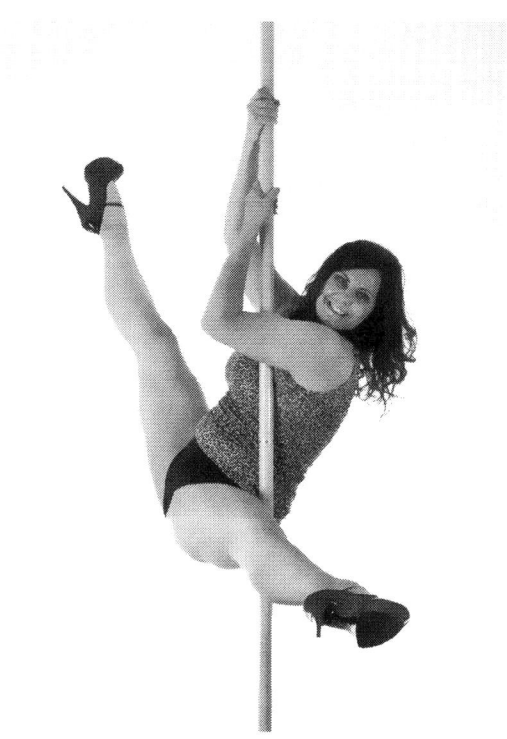

- Start standing to side of the pole
- Less dominant arm low, dominant arm high
- Step weight onto your outside foot
- Pull up and sweep the inside leg over (think cartwheel)
- Outside leg follows in the same pattern
- Keep body close to the pole
- Land gently on your feet
- Repeat on the other side

GSM's notes

"If you forget to pull up with this one, you will just sink down. It's all in the arms. The legs can be bent to start with if this is more comfortable for you, but you are eventually aiming to have beautifully elongated legs. Remember to point your feet."

Your notes:

_____
_____
_____
_____

Level Two

How exciting gorgeous one! You are progressing beautifully. Welcome to Level Two. This level introduces more spins, which now need a little more strength - both in your grip and your body.

Remember when practising all spins to gently step into each move and really use your arm strength to pull you upwards (in other words keep your shoulders down and back).

There will be new moves that transition from the climb and just a little word of warning - these are going to cause you some discomfort on your inner thighs. Don't worry it will get better.

Then finally, and this is where my students get very excited, you will be learning to invert. Please make sure you have a spotter on hand to help you in the beginning stages of any invert.

There is a natural progression of moves in Level Two and it will serve your body and safety well to learn and become confident in each move before moving on to the next. Especially when learning the inverts.

Have fun!

Level Two

Kiss

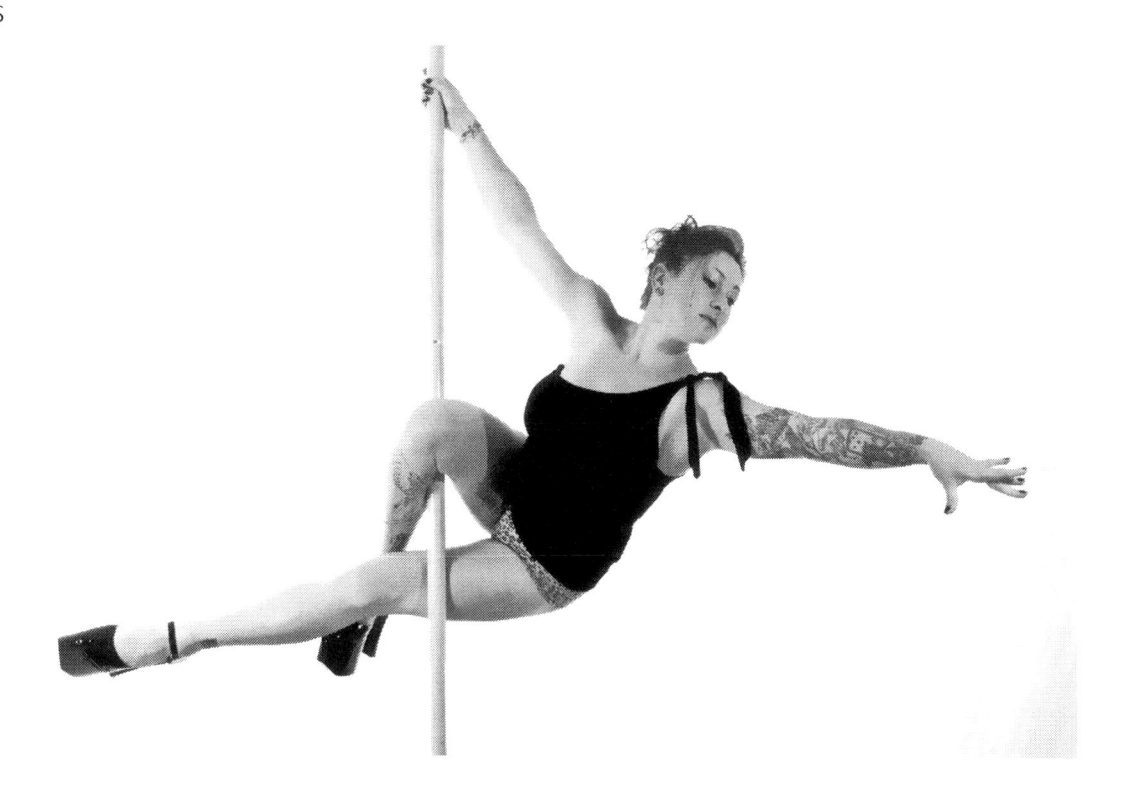

- Start standing side on to pole
- Dominant arm is high
- Weight is on your outside foot
- Lift and hook your inside leg up high on the pole
- Lead with hips as you lean forward
- Lift bottom leg off the floor and lift it so it is straight behind the pole
- Spin all the way to the floor, you will land on your side

GSM's notes

"The more you push your hips forward with this move, the more you will spin. Some girls get stuck halfway because they grip too much with the back of the knee. Putting on a pair of trousers always sorts that out! This works better with your dominant arm only on the pole but when teaching this, I encourage the girls to use both arms."

Your notes:

_____
_____
_____
_____

Level Two
Outside Tucks - Chair

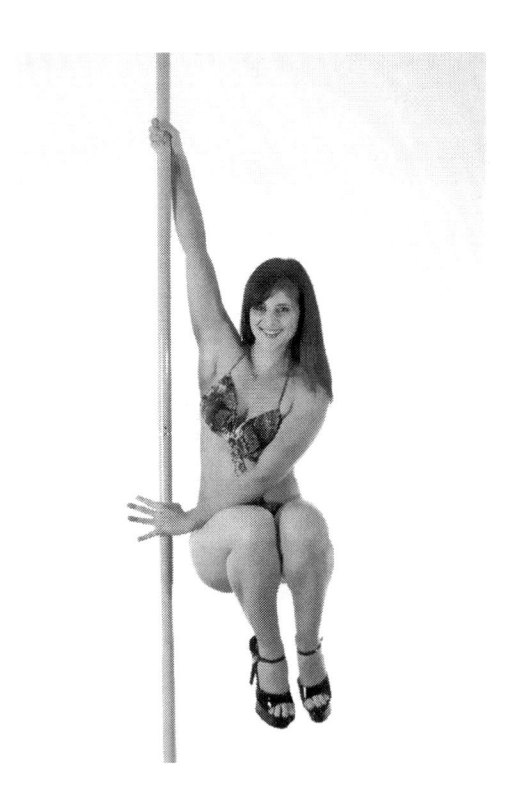

- Start standing side on to pole
- Dominant arm high, less dominant arm waist height as picture
- Step on inside foot, sweep outside leg around, whilst pulling up with your arms
- Draw knees up into your tummy using your abdominals and spin around
- Use the less dominant arm to control your position on the pole
- Land on feet and step out
- Repeat the other way

GSM's notes

"The Outside Tucks are a little harder as you are just relying on arm strength and momentum. The more I pull up on my top arm, the better this looks. Keep your knees together and toes pointed. Your Strength Tucks on page 33 will help you do this."

Your notes:
_____
_____
_____
_____

Level Two
Outside Tucks - Frog

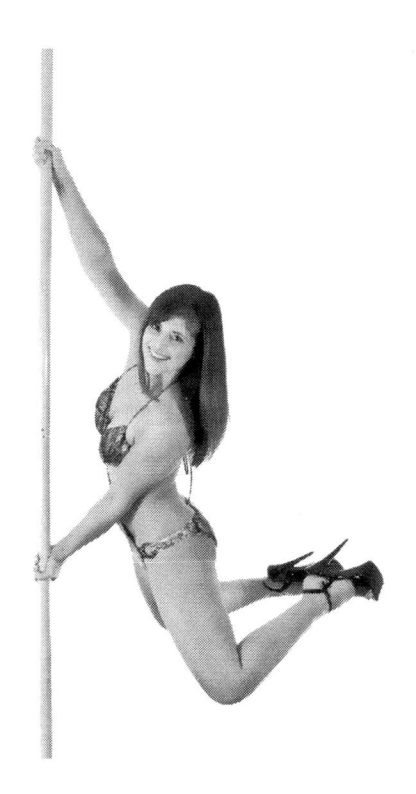

- Start side on to pole
- Dominant arm high
- Weight on the inside foot, sweep outside leg around
- Shoulders down, pull up with arm on pole
- Place less dominant arm, thumb and fingers pointing downwards on pole
- Keep your body lifted and strong - body will be facing the pole as you spin
- Bring heels together
- Spin to floor, land on knees
- Repeat the other way

GSM's notes

"The trick is to keep your body lifted and strong from the top of your head right down to your toes. Really pull up on your top arm too."

Your notes:

Level Two
Outside Tucks - V Spin

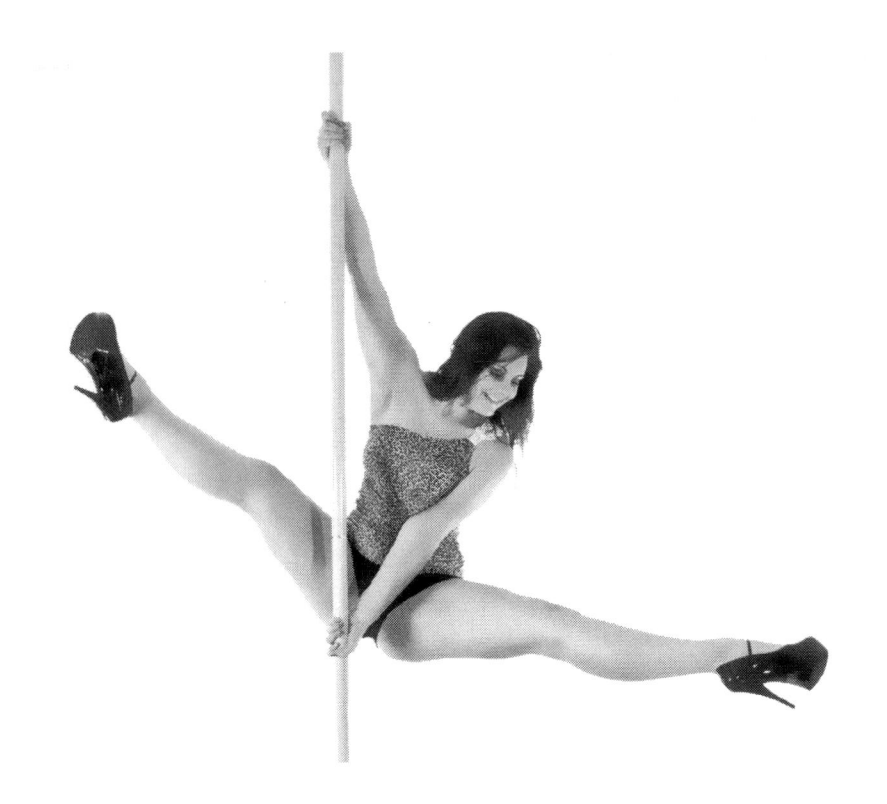

- Start standing side on to pole, dominant arm is high
- Weight is on the inside foot
- Sweep outside leg around
- Shoulders down, pull up through arms, placing outside hand, thumb and fingers pointing downwards, onto the pole
- Draw legs up as high as you comfortably can - use abdominals
- Bring feet into base of pole to finish this move
- Repeat the other way

GSM's notes

"When you work from your abdominals to lift your legs, this move gets a lot easier to do. Practise lifting your legs without the spin first so you can learn to isolate these muscles - a great strengthening move for you. Another tip is to practise this move with bent knees."

Your notes:
___
___
___
___

Level Two
Inside Tucks

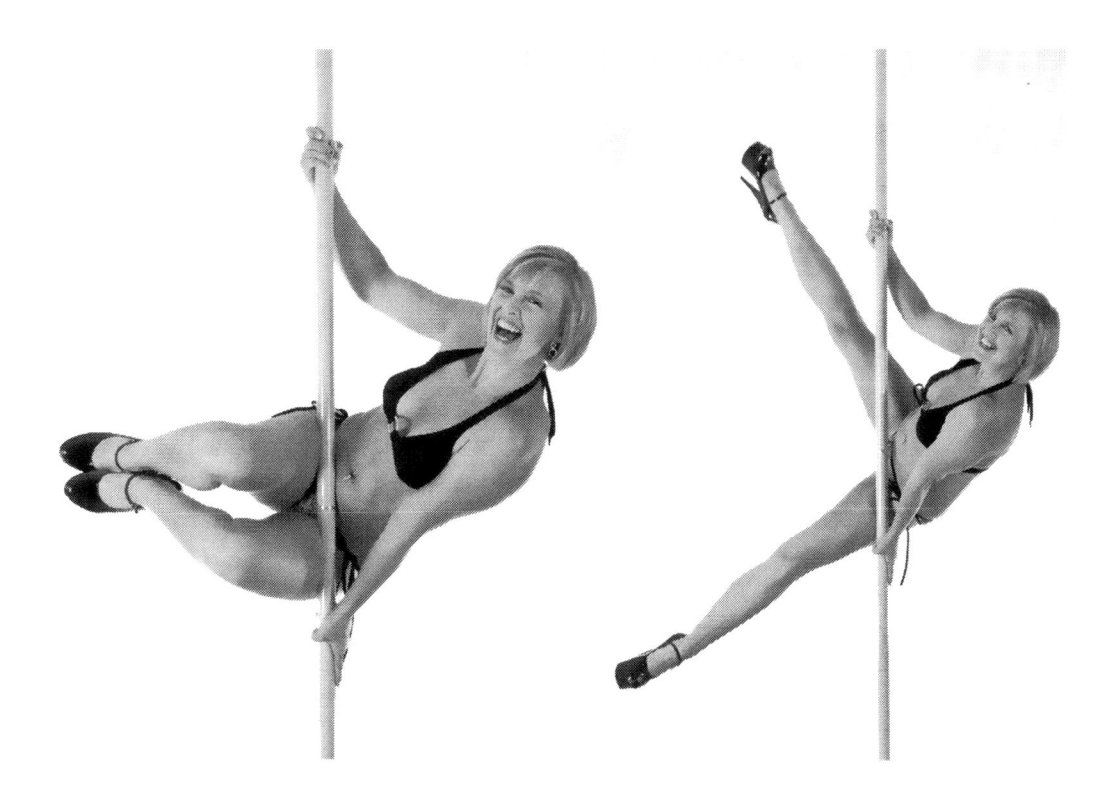

- Start this spin standing side on to the pole with your less dominant arm next to the pole
- Dominant arm head height
- Less dominant arm hip height with fingers and thumb facing downwards
- Weight is on your inside foot
- Sweep outside leg around
- Lift both knees into tummy as you lean your body away from legs - you can also open the legs into a V as in the 2nd picture
- The more you lean your body horizontally, the easier it is

GSM's notes

"A little confusing this one as you are spinning the other way! So once you have figured that out, you need to work with both arms (pulling with the top and pushing with the bottom) and the more horizontal you are the better this spin works."

Your notes:
_____
_____
_____
_____

Level Two
Mini Spins

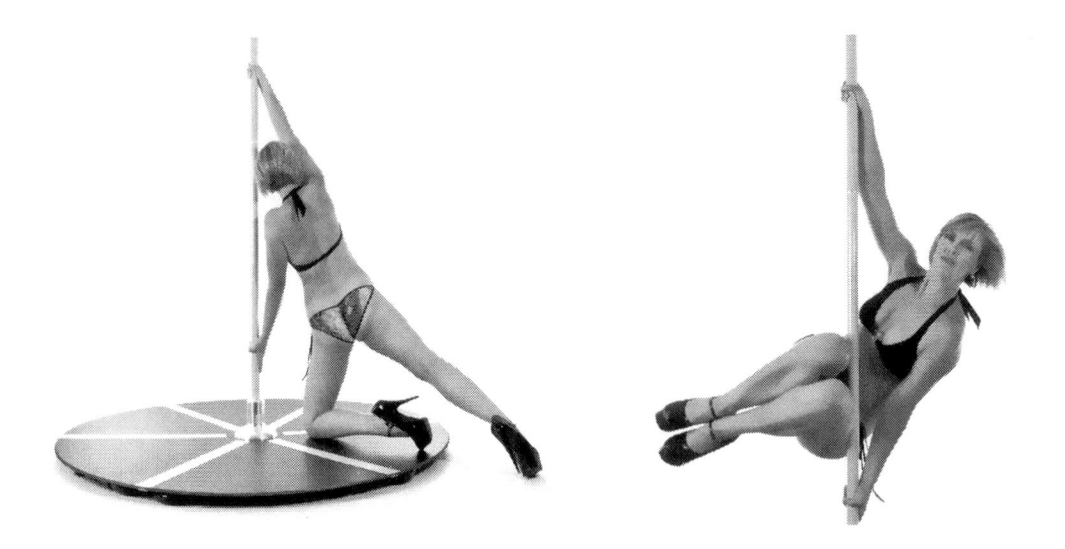

- This is exactly like the Inside Tucks on the previous page, but you start on your knees
- Great transition move from the floor to standing

GSM's notes

"I love this move as it helps you flow from one move to another. You can always do this move with the hands close together too – it's easier."

Your notes:
_____
_____
_____
_____

Level Two

Sunwheel

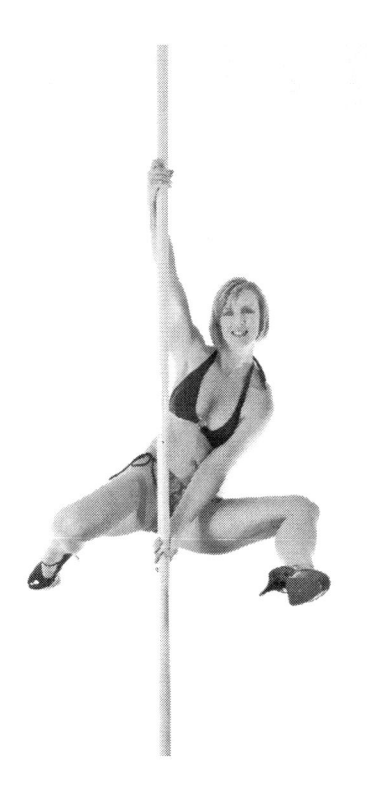

- My helpful tip - sit on the floor with your legs in an attitude position (as picture) to help get your orientation
- Standing side on to pole
- Dominant arm high
- Weight on inside foot
- Sweep outside leg around and lift up as per picture
- Place less dominant arm on pole hip height, fingers pointing down
- Shoulders down and back
- Lifting back leg up behind you
- Spin to floor, landing gently on your bottom

GSM's notes

"A sneaky leg workout - the more you lift from your abdominals and legs the better this looks. Pointing your feet will also make this one look fabulous!"

Your notes:
___
___
___
___

Level Two
Backwards Attitude

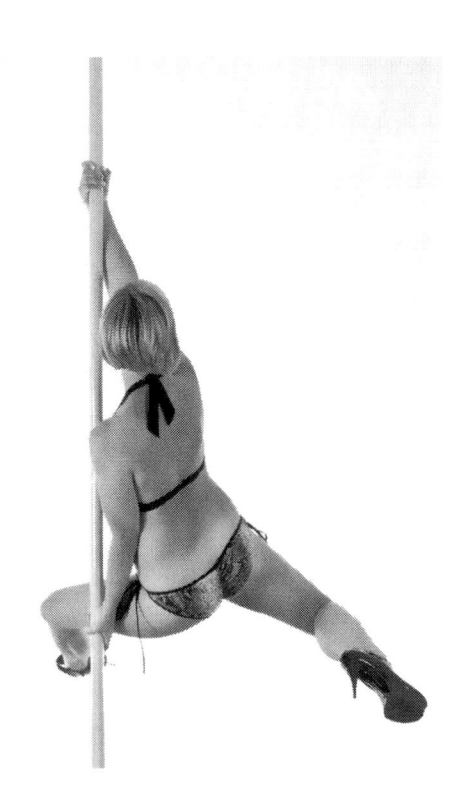

- My helpful tip - sit on the floor with your legs in an attitude position (as picture) to help get your orientation
- Start standing with your less dominant side to the pole
- Dominant arm high, less dominant arm low - thumb and fingers facing downwards
- Sweep outside leg backwards in a big circle
- Lift both legs into an attitude position
- Finish the spin by landing on the floor on your bottom
- Repeat on the other side

GSM's notes

"You can also do this spin with the inside hand at waist height - hugging the pole. Really use your muscles to lift your legs up and hold them. It makes this move look so graceful."

Your notes:

_____
_____
_____
_____

Level Two

One Arm Spiral

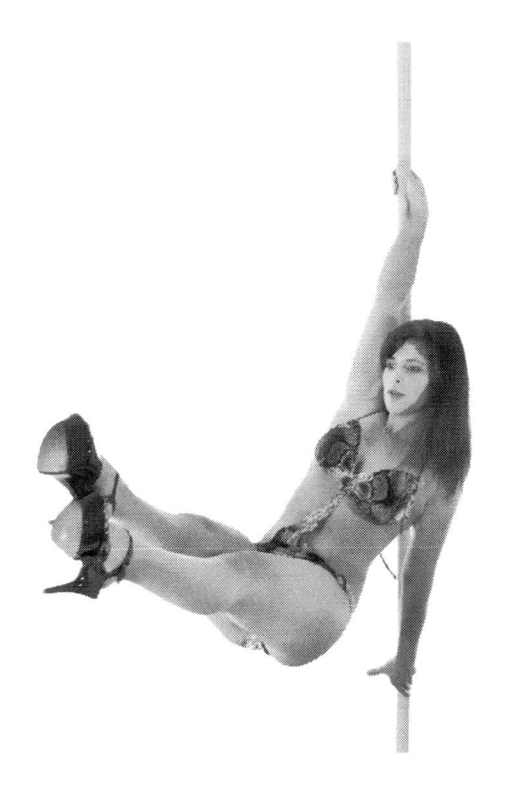

- Start with your back to the pole
- Take dominant arm high, wrap arm around the pole, fingers and thumb pointing upwards
- Less dominant arm on pole, thumb and fingers pointing downwards
- Shoulders down and back
- Extend inside leg out
- Lean away from the leg with the body
- Sweep inside leg around the pole lifting the other leg to spin
- You will spin with your back to the pole
- Land on your feet

GSM's notes

"Please note the picture above shows the full One Arm Spiral movement. I really need great grip for the full version of this spin, otherwise I end up flying across the other side of the room. It's all about strength and confidence, progress slowly and soon you will be performing the full version."

Your notes:

_____

_____

_____

_____

Level Two
Crucifix

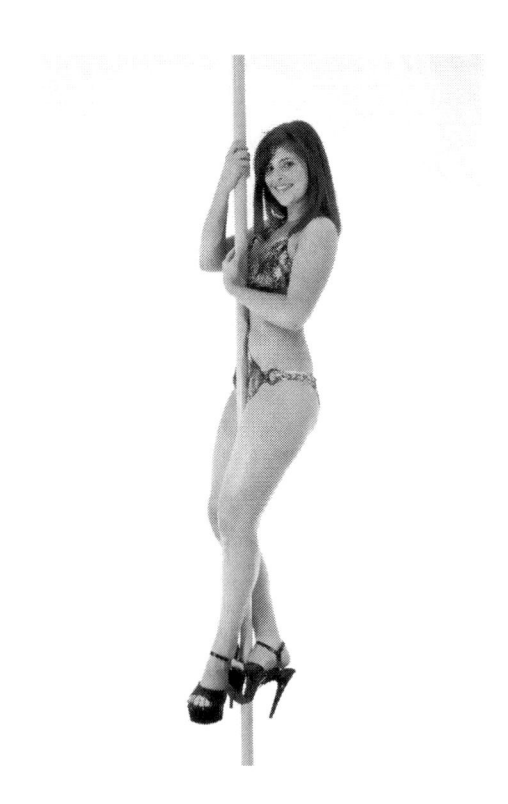

- As you spend more time on the pole, your arm strength will increase which helps your climbing technique
- Climb as in level one - page 25 and place the legs on the pole as above
- Slide elegantly down

GSM's notes

"As your strength improves there are so many options with climbing, you can spin, hold, and climb all the way to the top. Shoes or boots are great as they will help you stick to the pole."

Your notes:

_____
_____
_____
_____

Level Two

Layback

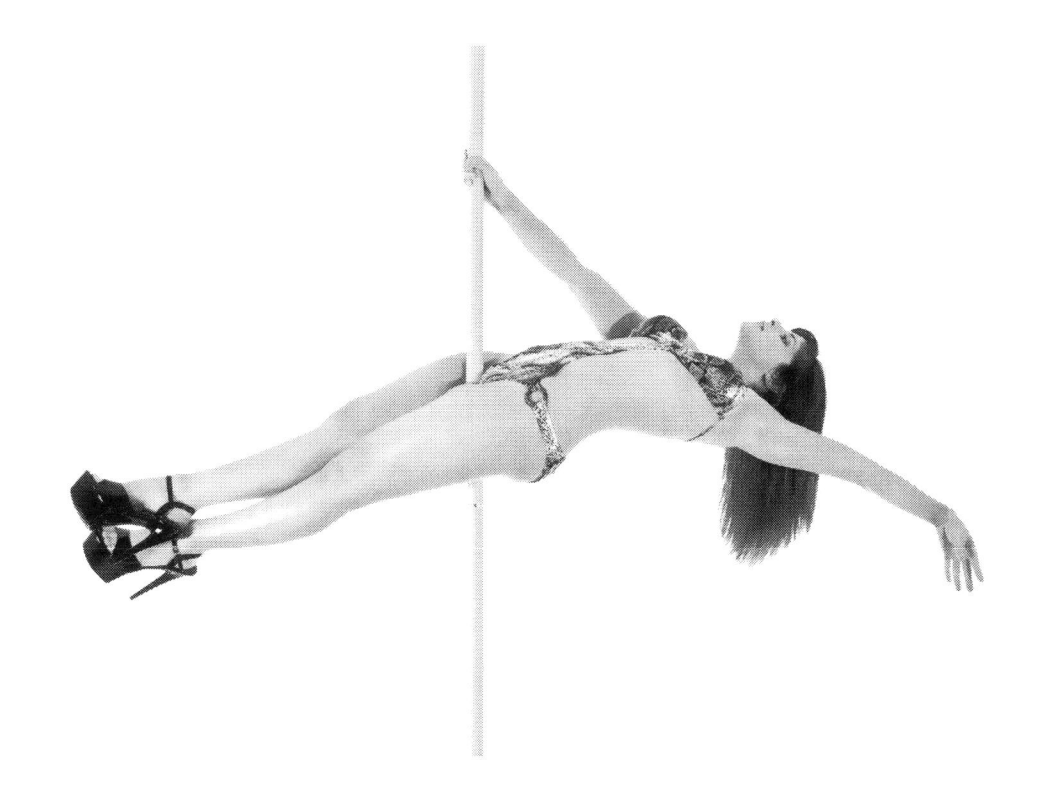

- This move works beautifully from your Goddess Sit (page 24)
- Extend both legs out straight and cross at your ankles
- Walk both hands down the pole
- Leave dominant arm on the pole
- Extend other arm out behind you
- Hold body strong and slightly push the legs down

GSM's notes

"Really extend your body and squeeze your bottom and legs to get a great shape to this move. You are getting a sneaky leg and butt workout here too!"

Your notes:
_____
_____
_____
_____

Level Two
Open for Business

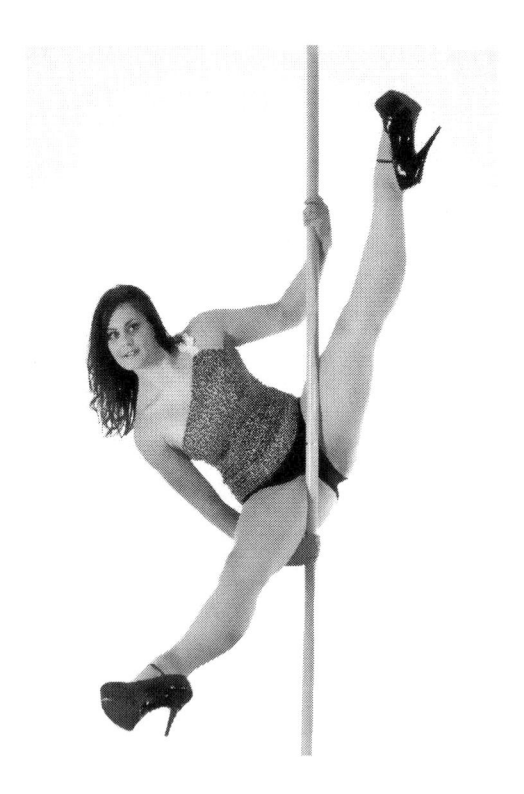

- From a Goddess Sit (page 24)
- Place less dominant arm underneath your bottom, thumb and fingers pointing upwards
- Angle body towards this arm
- Lean slightly to the side
- Open your legs
- Pole will be sitting underneath your bottom sitting bone

GSM's notes

"The more I tilt my pelvis in the Goddess Sit before, the more comfortable this move is. This will take a little practice and you may slide but remember to pull your shoulders down and lift your chest."

Your notes:

_____
_____
_____
_____

Level Two
Goddess

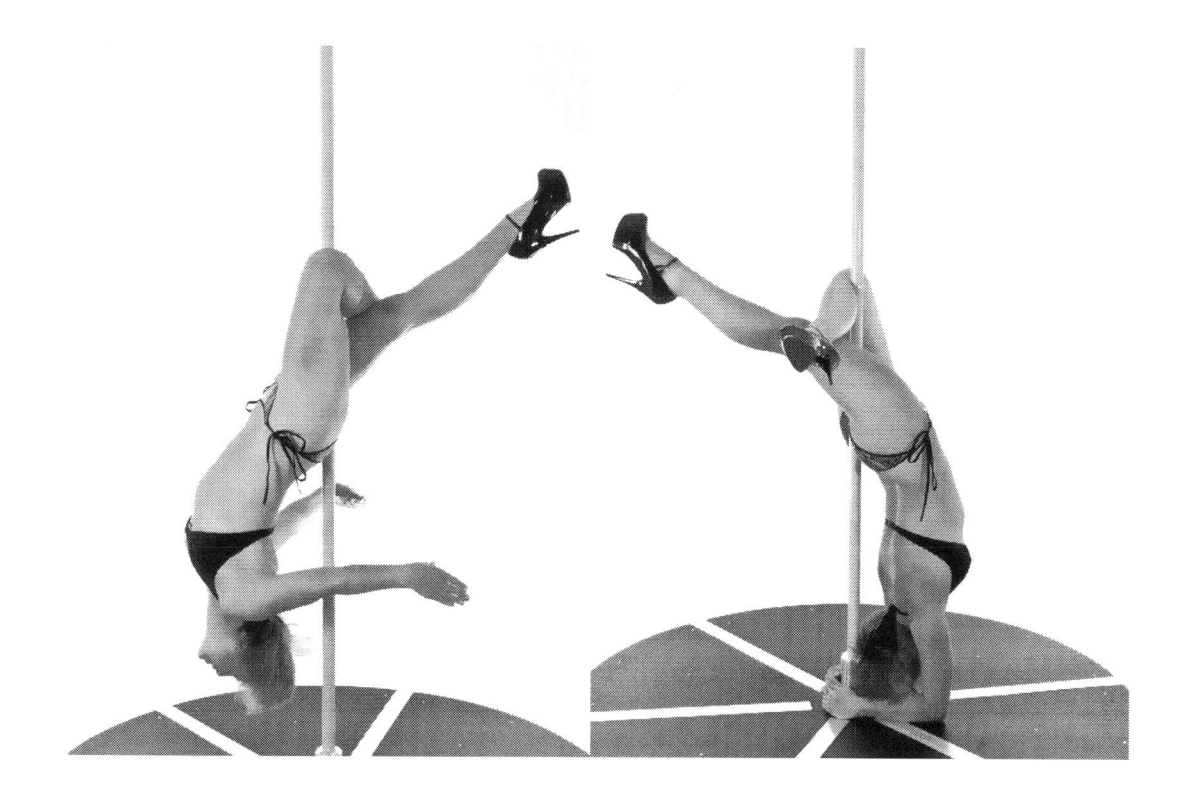

- From a Goddess Sit (page 24)
- Walk both hands down pole and lean body backwards
- Lift both legs up, the pole will sit into the crease of the top knee - make sure you are pushing the bottom leg up to the ceiling
- Your next stage is to hold this position. When secure, you can release hands and hold this - a great abdominal workout
- As you build your confidence up, you can lower yourself all the way down and hang
- Options out of the Goddess - return to sitting (abdominal strength) or go down into a headstand as above or handstand (not shown)

GSM's notes

"Please use a spotter when starting out in this move - this will help your confidence and safety. The more you push your bottom leg up to the ceiling, the more stable you become on the pole. Trust me, your thighs will get used to the pain!"

Your notes:

_____
_____
_____
_____

Level Two
Basic Invert

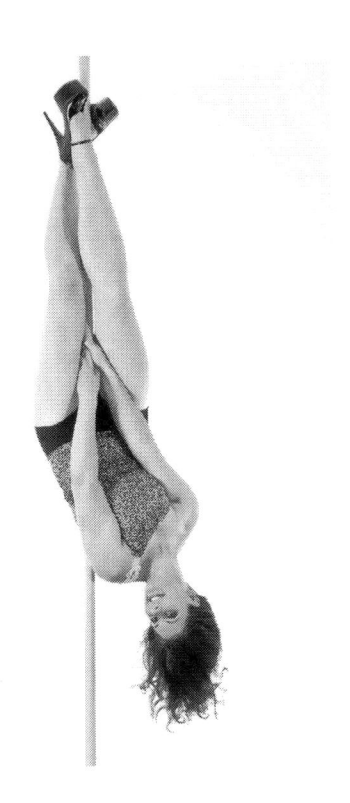

- Standing with your less dominant side to the pole
- Less dominant arm chest height, hugging pole
- Dominant arm chin height
- Focus your eyes on the pole where the legs are going which is just above your hands
- Weight on inside foot
- Sweep outside leg upwards - you are aiming this leg to go in front of the pole - so the back of the ankle rests on the pole (I'm using the orientation as if you are upside down)
- The inside leg follows contacting the back of the pole with the front of the foot
- Lean body back as your legs go up - this move is more about leaning backwards than inverting
- Grip with your thighs and feet
- Slide down to floor on your back
- Strength option: I teach my girls to reverse dismount too. This takes a lot of control and is an excellent conditioning move.

GSM's notes

"It's all about focus - you need to focus on where your leg is going to go on the pole, think about tilting back rather than going upside down. Girls always smile BIG when they get this one!"

Your notes:

_____
_____
_____
_____

Level Two
Inverted Crucifix

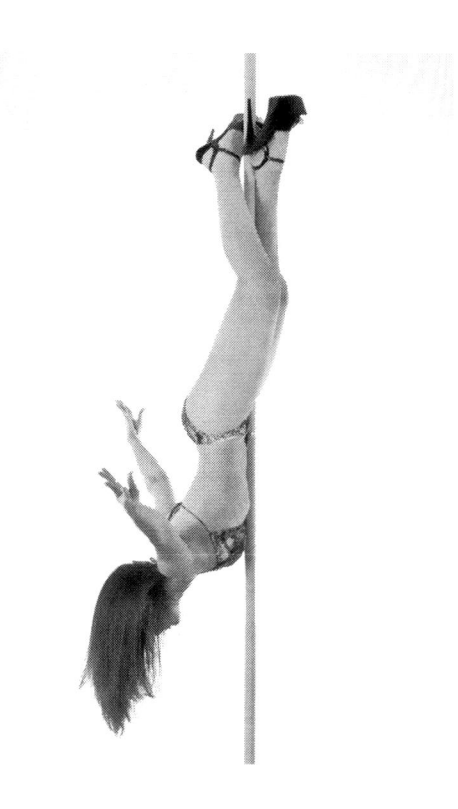

- From invert, legs are long up the pole gripping with your thighs
- Your pubic bone is touching the pole
- Take your less dominant arm off and replace underneath your head
- Rotate your body towards the pole
- Take your dominant arm down and replace underneath your head
- When your confidence increases you can remove both hands
- To exit, slide down into Handstand, see page 52, and step off

GSM's notes

"A spotter is essential when starting out. It's all in the thighs – roll them together and squeeze the pole. Take this one slowly."

Your notes:
_____
_____
_____
_____

Level Two

Handstand from Inverted Crucifix

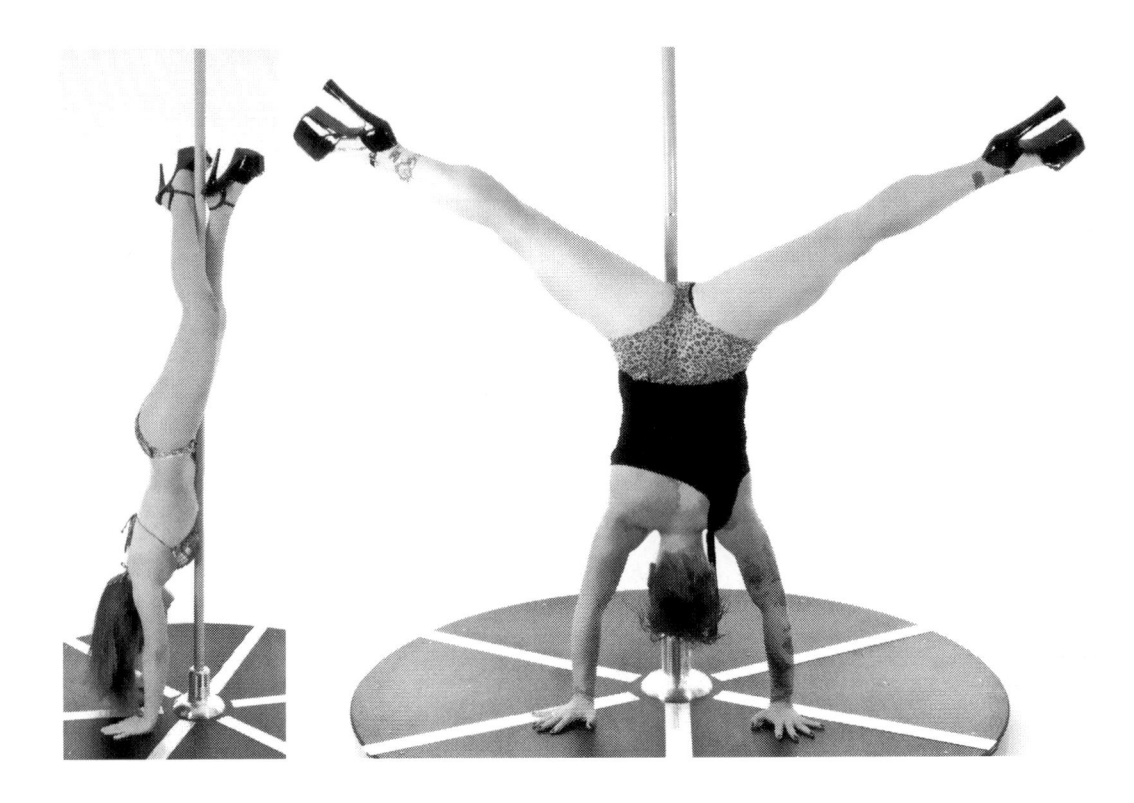

- Hands underneath your shoulders, shoulder distance apart
- Shoulders rotated down and back
- Abdominals in
- Think long through your body
- You can open the legs into a V - press your belly into the pole to help you balance

GSM's notes

"I advise my girls to practise handstands against the wall, so they understand what muscles have to work to hold you here. Shoulders down and back, and remember this is going to be super challenging as we have all our weight going down into our arms. Rest your belly on the pole and think about lengthening up to the sky. To come out, you can walk the hands forward and slide the legs down so you end up on your belly. Or just step your leg down then the other to the side of the pole."

Your notes:

_____
_____
_____
_____

Level Two
Outside Leg Hook

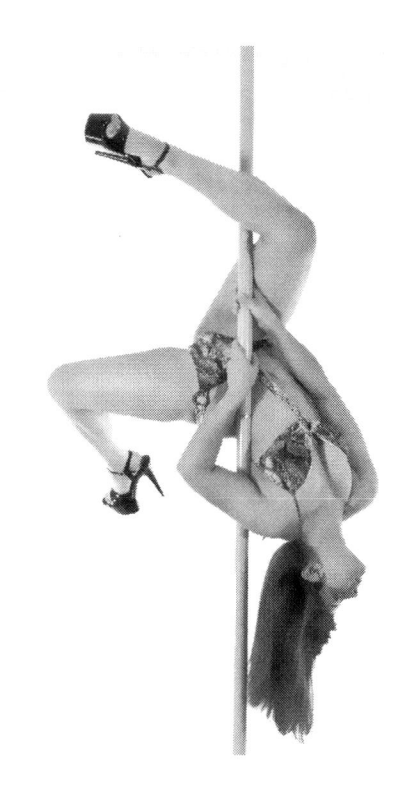

- From a Basic Invert with both legs on the pole - page 50
- Slide outside leg down the pole and bend the knee so the pole sits into the back of the knee - need to grip with the leg to hold this
- Make sure the toes are pointing down to the floor (NB Julia is doing a slightly different version here)
- Other leg extends away from the body to balance you - bent or straight
- Options when secure - remove top hand off first, followed by the bottom hand

GSM's notes

"The more you keep your pelvis close to the pole, the easier this move is to do. It's all about getting the right grip with the outside leg."

Your notes:
_____
_____
_____
_____

Level Two

Straddle Preps into Full Straddle

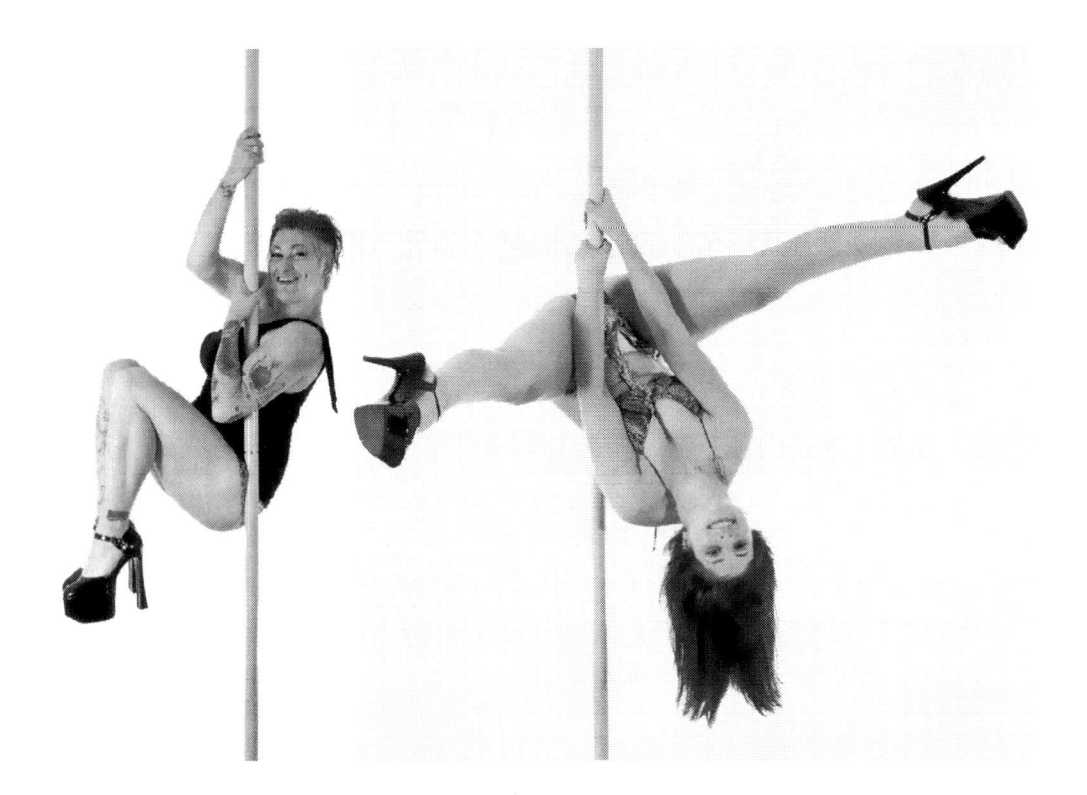

- To start, practise your Tucks (page 33) to the same side as you would invert using control back down
- Then Tuck and tilt your body backwards (no picture shown) - this is going to be a challenge
- As your strength increases, from the tilt back you can extend the legs over your head into a Straddle - point your feet and elongate the legs
- Keep your pubic bone close to the pole
- Lower down with control

GSM's notes

"Super arm and abdominal strength - here you come! Practice makes perfect with this one. Once you have got it, then you can spin this lovely move too. Oh, and then you can practise on the other side."

Your notes:

_____
_____
_____
_____

Level Three

From strength comes confidence - confidence in yourself and on and around the pole. As your strength and confidence increases, welcome to Level Three.

Your 'basic' spin collection is completed by the Flying Squirrel and now, this level is all about expanding your aerial skills on the pole and teaching you a greater variety of transitions from climbs and inverting, which will all need great strength. So, please make sure you have nailed the inverts in Level Two before progressing here.

As you meander through Level Three, a lot of my students feel they plateau and do get frustrated. I'm sure that throughout your pole training, you have noticed that one week you can execute your moves perfectly and the next week nothing seems to go right. Well, the answer to this is that when we learn any new complex movement or sequence it can take up to 10 years or 1,000,000 repetitions to make it automatic to our bodies. So, please have patience and know that everything will fall into place when your body is ready.

If you have a pole at home, I would suggest that you practise 2 - 3 x per week for about 30 - 40 mins, using my formula in the essential tricks and tips section.

Personally, I practise Pilates and weight train x 3 per week. This, entwined with my pole dancing practice, really does help me become stronger on and off the pole.

Don't forget your spotter, chalk, towel and an attention to your posture - and you are off...

Level Three
Invert to Vertical

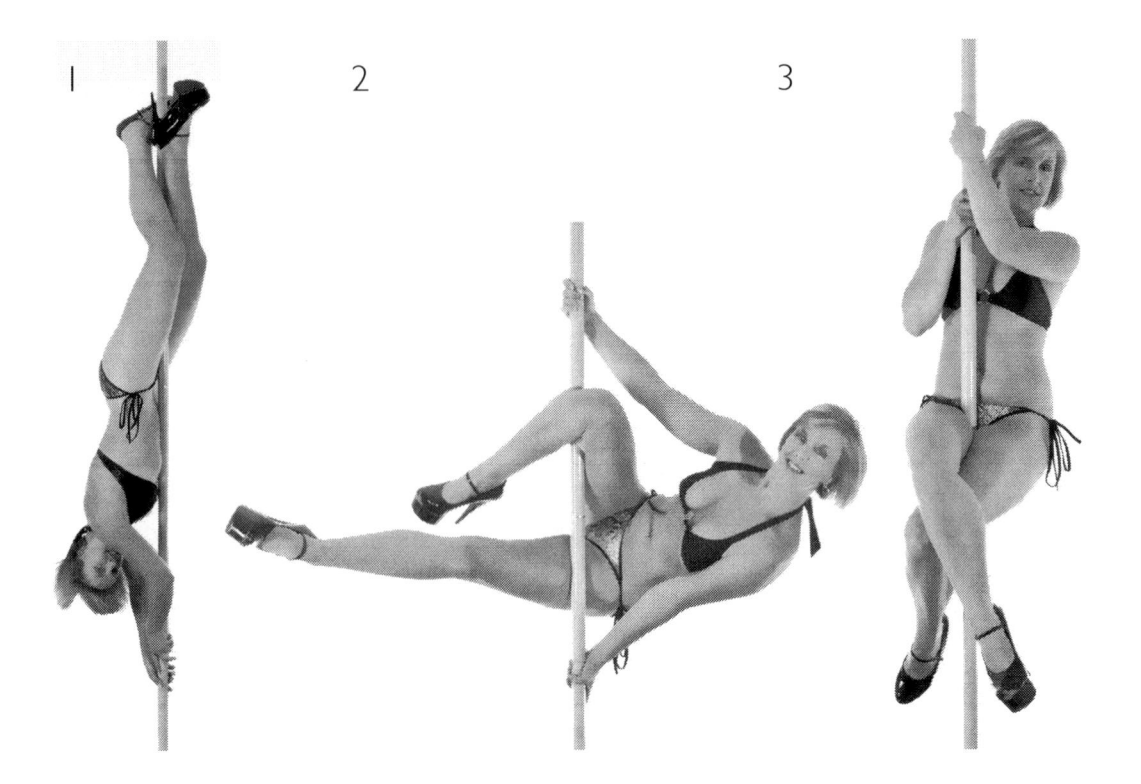

1   2   3

- Basic Invert (page 50) and move into an Inverted Crucifix (picture 1)
- Move in to an Outside Leg Hook (page 53)
- Take dominant arm and place above your hooked leg - you will need great grip on your hooked leg and abdominal strength
- Replace less dominant arm lower down and hold (picture 2)
- Replace less dominant arm above the hooked leg so you can pull yourself upright
- Then whilst pulling up with the arms legs slide down and cross to sit on pole, (picture 3)

GSM's notes

"This is an essential combination to get you from inverted to vertical. It takes some practice and once you have nailed it there are so many moves you can do from this."

Your notes:

_____
_____
_____
_____

Level Three

Princess

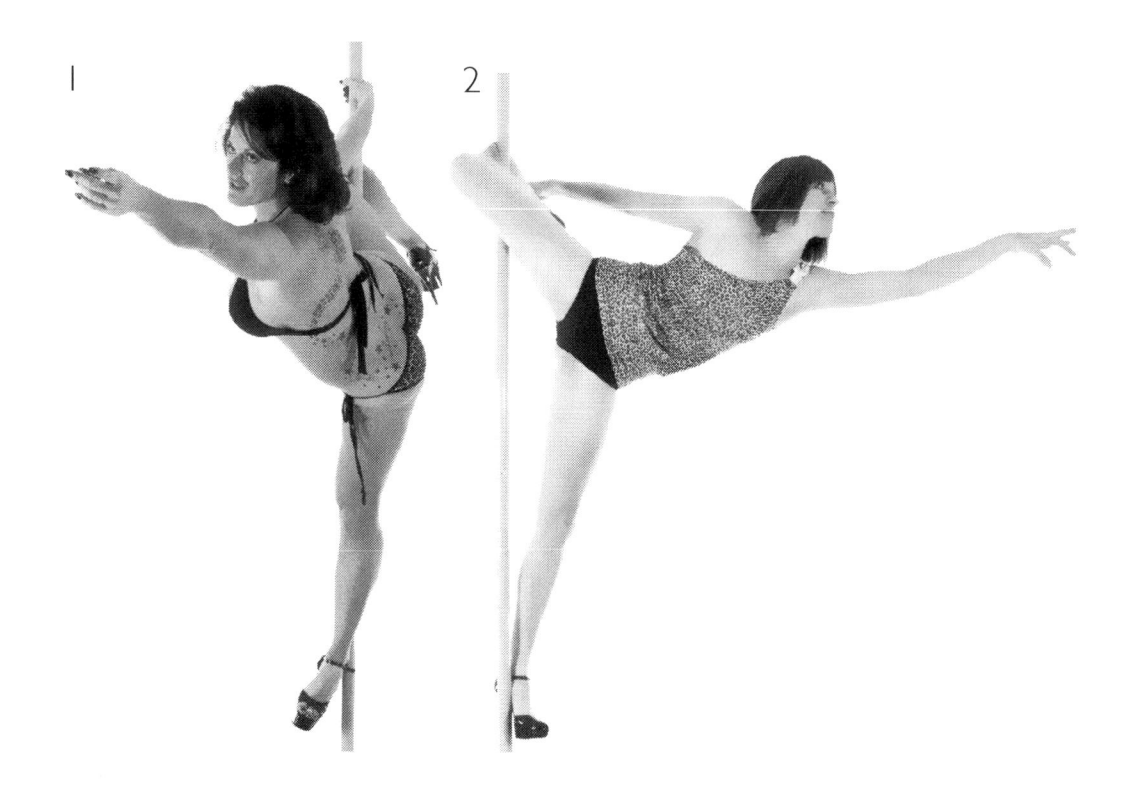

- Basic Invert (page 50) and move into an Inverted Crucifix (page 51)
- Move into position 2 of your Invert to Vertical (page 56)
- Take inside leg down the pole and rest to the side as above or tuck the foot behind pole
- Making sure you have great grip on the back of your hooked knee and the foot is pointing down to the floor take your body parallel to the floor
- You can now either hold above the top leg (picture 1) or pull your top heel towards your bottom with your dominant arm (picture 2), and extend less dominant arm out.

GSM's notes

"This is all about the grip you have with your top leg. Sometimes I just can't grip and other times it is perfect. A little chalk behind your knee can help."

Your notes:

_____
_____
_____
_____

Level Three

Showgirl / Star

1   2

Showgirl   Star

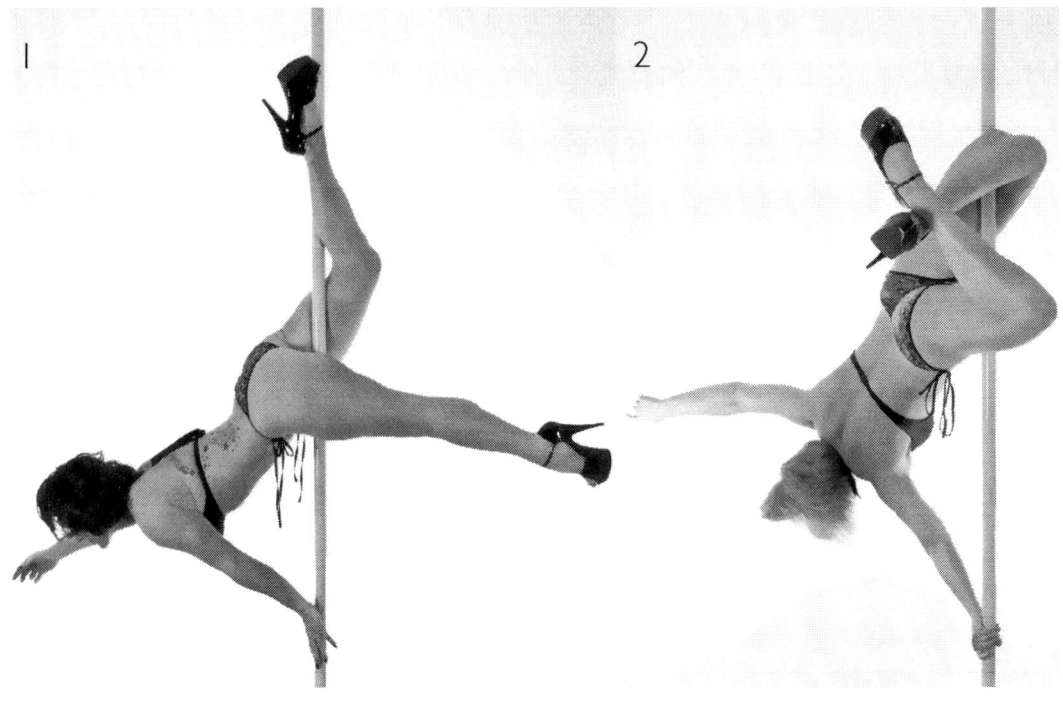

- Invert to Outside Leg Hook (page 53)
- Move into position 2 of your Invert to Vertical (page 56)
- Bring your unhooked leg in towards the pole so toes are pointing down to the floor
- Squeeze inner thighs around the pole
- You can place your less dominant arm on the pole underneath your legs to help you stay secure
- Take your dominant arm off the pole and rotate your pelvis down to the floor whilst squeezing the pole with your hooked leg to prevent slipping
- Elongate your body out - as picture 1 and extend dominant arm out
- To go into your Star (2), bend the bottom knee and cross ankle - note your body will be turned to the side more on this move

GSM's notes

"I love these pretty moves and once you have mastered these, they are great in various combinations up the pole. Don't underestimate how much you need the grip and strength of your legs."

Your notes:

_____
_____
_____
_____

Level Three
Butterfly

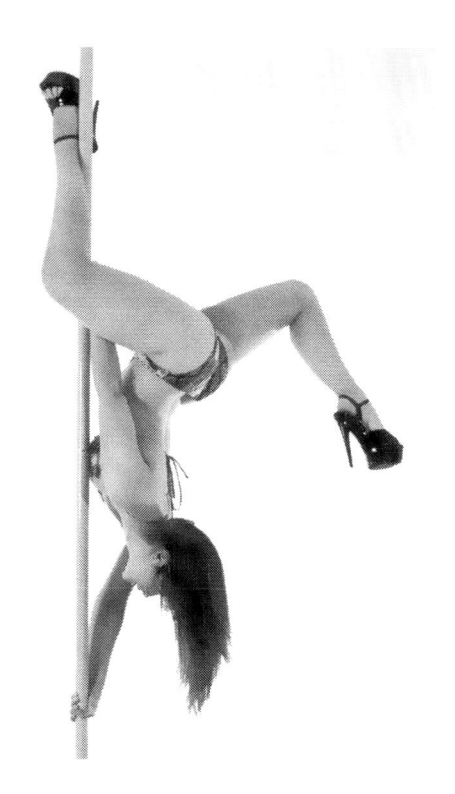

- Invert to an Inverted Crucifix (page 51)
- Less dominant arm goes down the pole, thumb and fingers face downwards, and re-grip
- Pull up with your dominant arm and push with your less dominant arm
- Make sure your body is lined up with the pole, with the top of your head pointing directly down to the floor
- Make sure your body is strong and stable, lengthen out through your sitting bones to the ceiling
- Then without dropping down - take back leg off pole and bend knee

GSM's notes

"*If I place my bottom hand slightly higher up the pole it pushes me out and up so I am further away from the pole - making this move look even better.*"

Your notes:

_____
_____
_____
_____

Level Three

Superman

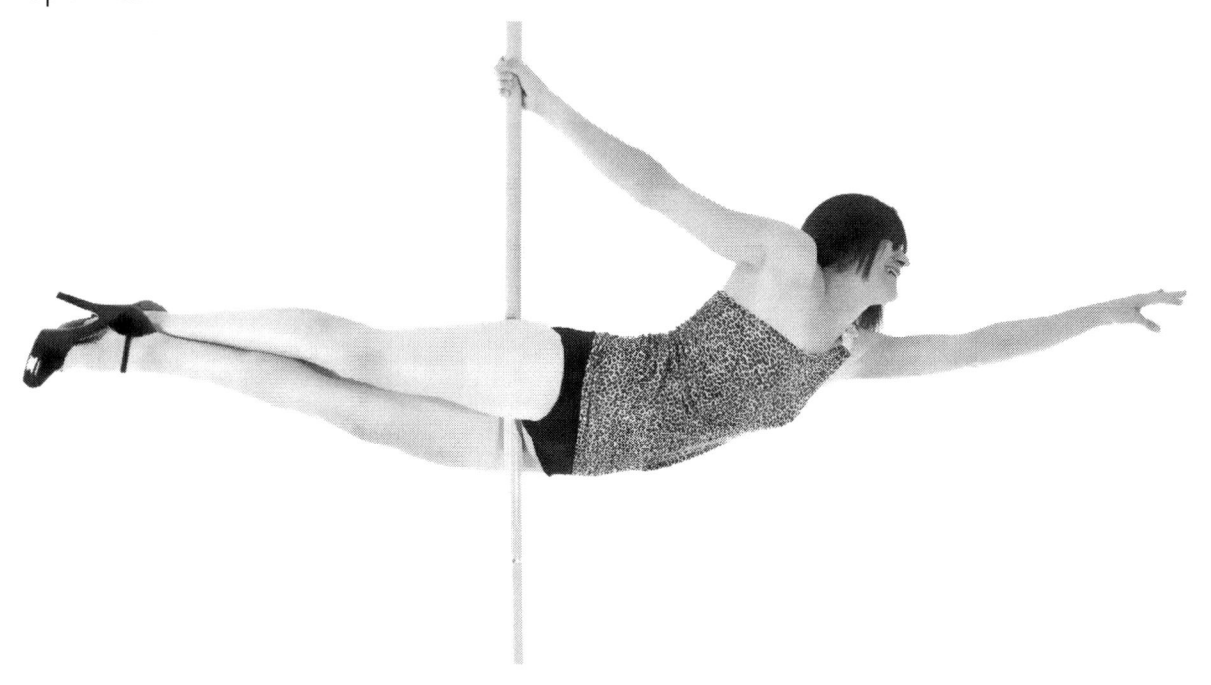

- Invert to Outside Leg Hook (page 53)
- Move in to position 2 of your Invert to Vertical (page 56)
- Pull up with your dominant arm whilst pushing against the pole with your less dominant arm
- Release the grip with your top leg and quickly rotate pelvis downwards
- Pull up with your dominant arm, extend legs out and cross them at your ankles, whilst releasing your less dominant arm
- Squeeze your legs together and extend less dominant arm out
- Pole will sit in between your inner thighs

GSM's notes

"Pain!!! Here it comes - this is super painful on your inner thighs when you are learning. It took me a while to nail this. I realised I had to really use my arm strength to help me twist my hips into this."

Your notes:

_____
_____
_____
_____

Level Three

Shoulder Mount

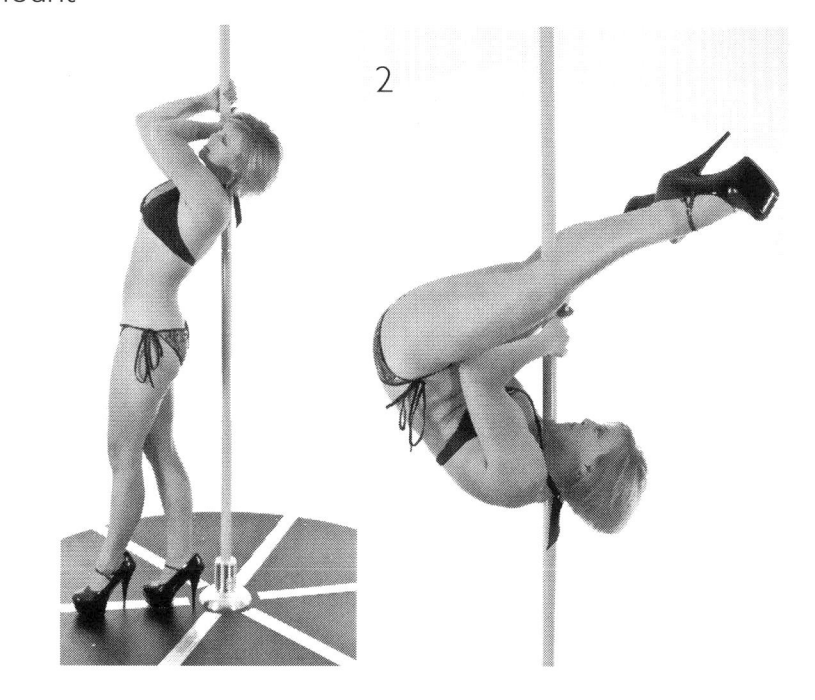

| 1 | 2 |

- Start with your back to pole, pole is resting in-between your spine and your shoulder blade on your dominant side (picture 1)
- Head to the other side of the pole, looking slightly up
- Both hands onto pole into a cupping grip
- Draw your elbows forward and down whilst keeping your shoulders down and back
- Chest up and abdominals are switched on
- To start the Shoulder Mount, here are 2 preps to help you:
  - Prep 1: Keeping the same height, draw your knees into your tummy hold and then release with control
  - Prep 2 - The next step is to tuck and tilt and release with control
- Then as your strength increases add a Straddle over your head as per picture 2 above
- You are aiming to keep the body in the same position without dropping
- Lower down with control

GSM's notes

"Options to come out - dismount with control or go into an Inverted Crucifix (page 51). Practise, practise, practise. Most of my girls took a long time to get this move. It needs a lot of strength and stability in your arms and core. Make sure you look up when placing the legs on the pole so you know where they are in space. Don't worry if you can't do it - all the time you are practising you are getting stronger."

Your notes:

_____
_____
_____
_____

Level Three

Straight Leg Climb

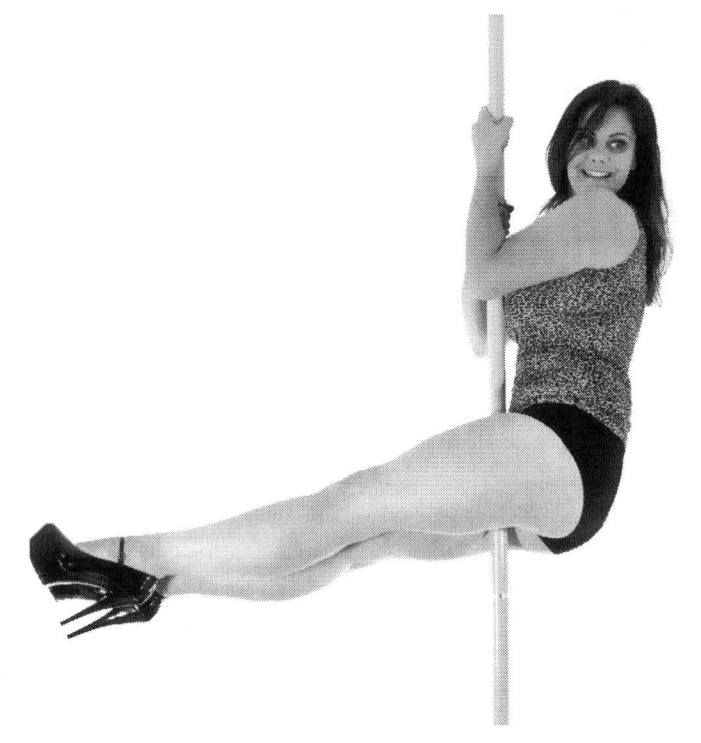

- This is an awesome conditioning move
- Climb up with arms only, legs stay out in front
- Repeat to come down

GSM's notes

"Uber strength move coming your way! A couple of times up and down the pole every session should do it! Great for all over body conditioning."

Your notes:
_____
_____
_____
_____

Level Three
Aerial Half Bracket Hold

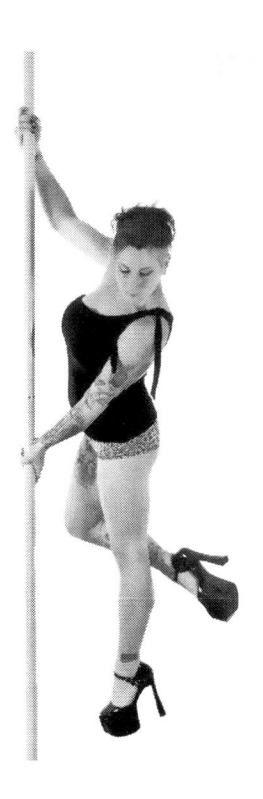

- Climb up the pole
- Keep you legs extended down the pole
- Split arms wide - dominant arm on top, less dominant arm below, grip as per picture
- Whilst pulling with dominant arm and pushing with less dominant arm take body away from the pole
- Options - you can take your legs into a V here too - replace your legs carefully back onto pole to exit

GSM's notes

"The more you pull up with the dominant arm the more control you get with this move. Be careful as you come out of this move not to just drop, always go in and out of your moves with control."

Your notes:

_____
_____
_____
_____

Level Three

Aerial Invert

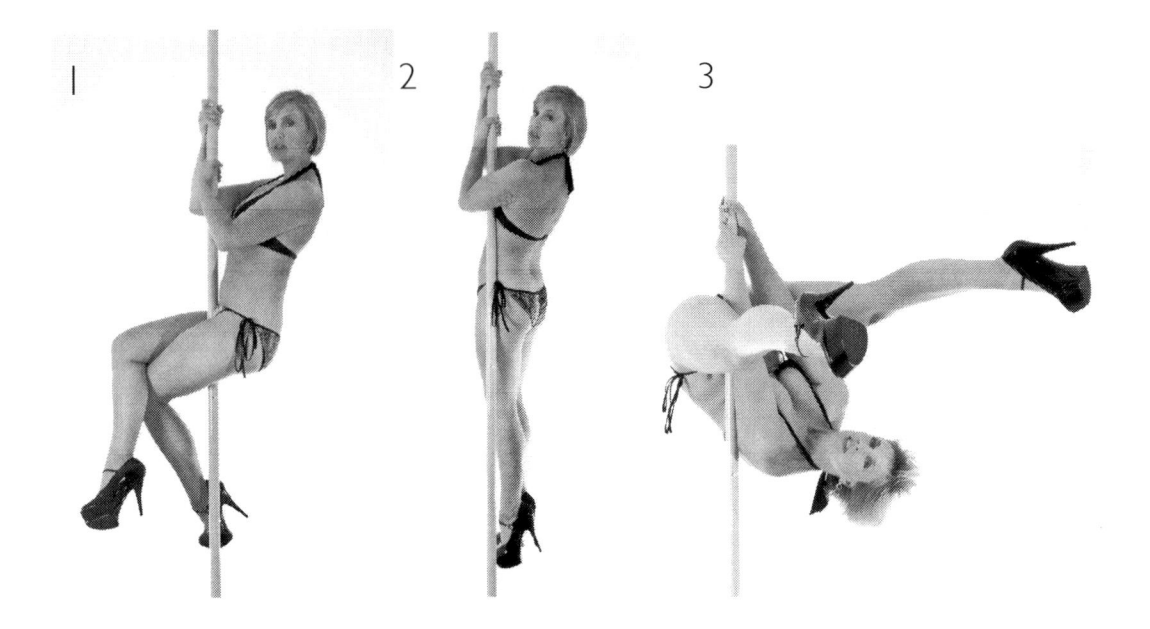

- Climb and sit (picture 1)
- Come to side of the pole - the same side you normally invert on (picture 2)
- Keep elbows bent - dominant arm on top, less dominant arm underneath
- Tuck and then invert
- Options to Basic Invert or Straddle (picture 3) or any of the Leg Hooks

GSM's notes

"This is a super strong move and a great transition move. You know you are strong when you can do this. If this is challenging for you, please do all the above but instead of inverting just Tuck and lower with control. You can do reps of 3-5 to build up your strength."

Your notes:

_____
_____
_____
_____

Level Three
Inside Leg Hook

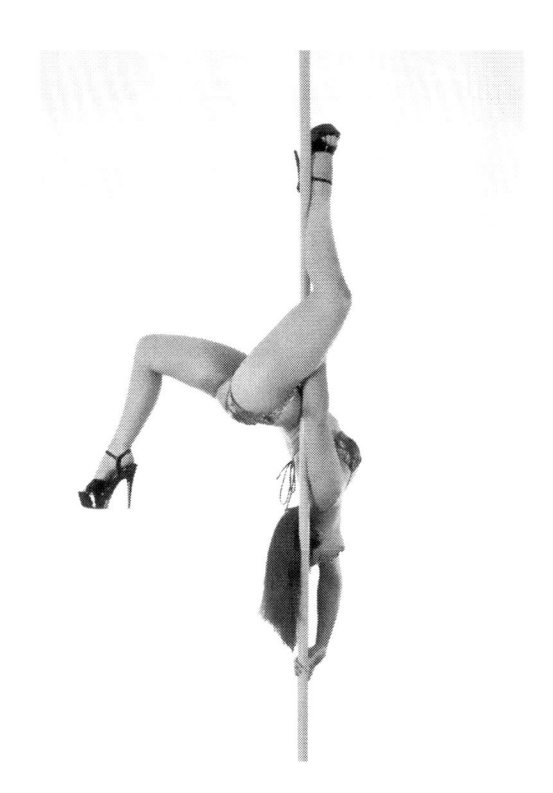

- Invert to Straddle (page 54)
- Inside leg hooks onto the pole as per above picture
- Get used to the feeling that you can hold your body with the leg
- Squeeze your inner thigh towards the pole
- Take other leg away from body opening out from your hip
- Keep your head up whilst you learn the orientation of your legs
- Pole sits in your waist
- Dominant arm goes low, less dominant arm stays in position
- Straddle out
- Option - can take your arms off the pole (needs grip)

GSM's notes

"Getting the pole to sit right in your waist will help you nail this move. Also getting the inside leg right around the pole and resist holding on with your foot so you can build up the strength in your legs to hold you here. Looks great."

Your notes:

_____
_____
_____
_____

Level Three
Advanced Layback

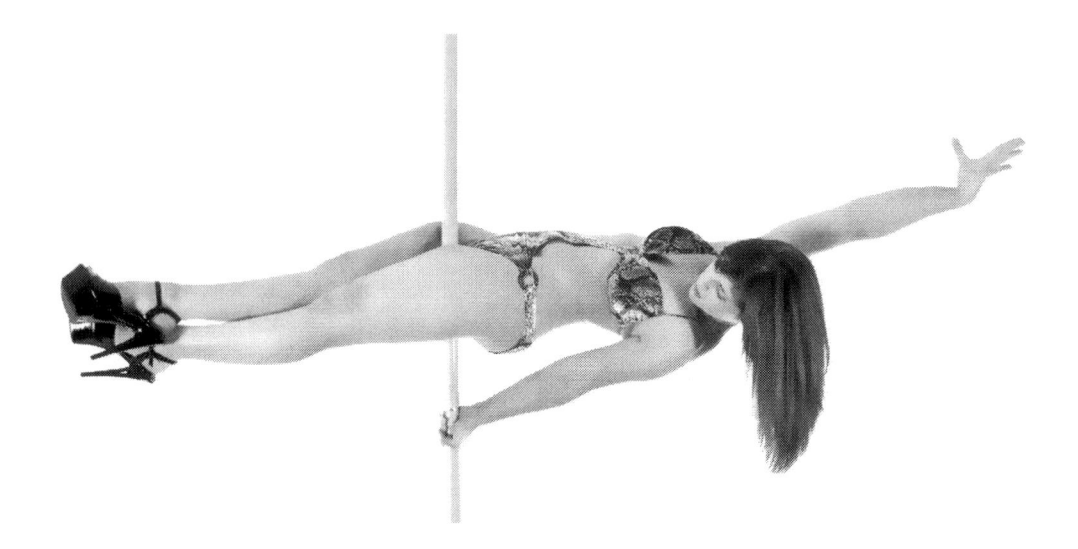

- As the Layback in Level 2 (page 47)
- Place your less dominant arm underneath you, thumb and fingers facing downwards
- Brace with this arm, shoulders down and back
- Extend top arm out whilst extending legs out
- Slightly push legs downwards, hips up and voila - hold!

GSM's notes

"Your body needs to tighten up and the more you push your hips to the ceiling the more stable you become. It may take a few tries but persevere."

Your notes:
_____
_____
_____
_____

Level Three

Flying Squirrel Spin

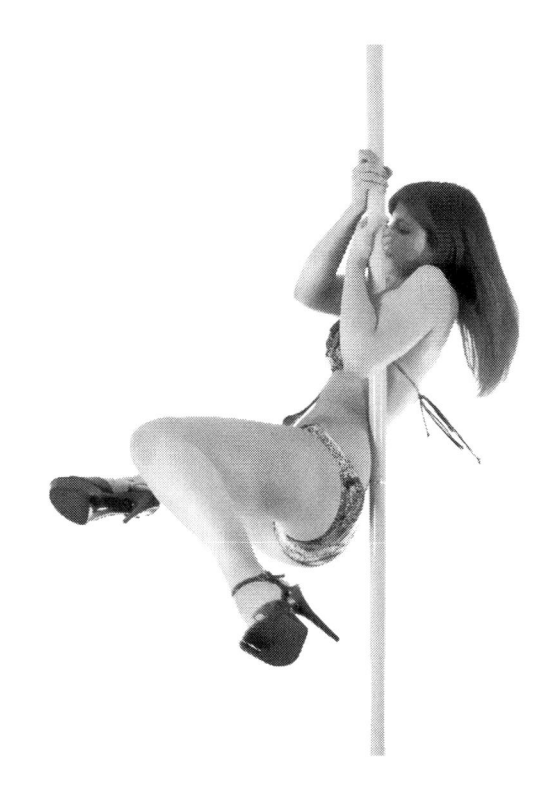

- Start in the same position as you would for the Inside Tuck (page 41)
- Less dominant arm shoulder height, dominant arm above head
- Weight is on your outside foot
- As you pull up through your arms keeping shoulders down...
- Sweep inside leg around, followed by the outside pulling legs up into an attitude position
- Spin with your back to the pole

GSM's notes

"I love this spin, the more I pull up before I go into my spin the better it looks, you can finish on your feet or on the floor".

Your notes:

_____
_____
_____
_____

Level Three
Lady Garden

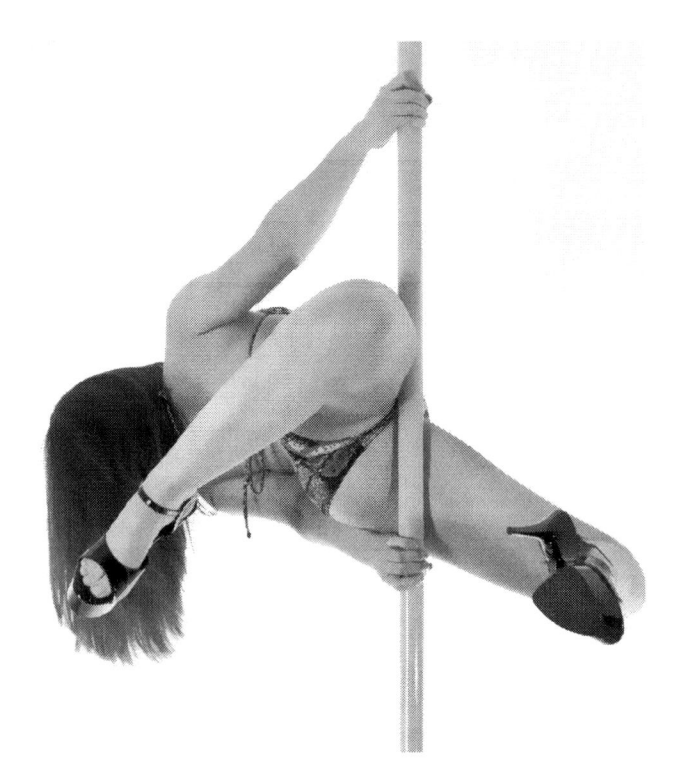

- Start as in Open for Business (page 48) but less dominant arm is thumb and forefinger pointing down
- Then arch back
- Bend the legs into an attitude position as per picture

GSM's notes

"I find this one quite hard to do as I have a really long back, Julia is demonstrating this beautifully. Really arch through your upper back to do this move."

Your notes:
_____
_____
_____
_____

Level Four

When strength and confidence come together, you just can't help it! You become sexy, you feel sexy and goddamit woman, you are sexy.

Enter Level Four. You are now mastering your own body with the skills you have learnt on the pole. Doesn't it feel good to be strong and in control of your own body all whilst having the best fun!

Level Four pushes you to achieve so much more and I have designed this level to challenge your strength and mind / body connection (you are going to need to be fearless).

The Level Four moves flow effortlessly from level three and again you really need to master level three before dipping your beautifully manicured toes into this level.

With patience, strength, practice and dedication trust me these moves will be yours.

By no means is the list of moves in my book the end, but by following these levels you are guaranteed to become stronger that you EVER thought possible and become a kick-arse pole dancer in the process!

The possibilities are endless with pole dancing with new moves and combinations being invented all the time.
Enjoy your body on and off the pole and believe that anything is possible! xxx

Level Four
Straight Leg Release

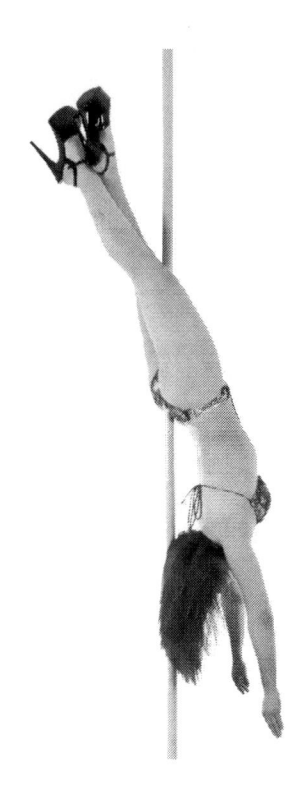

- Climb and sit (page 25) with your arms on the pole - dominant arm is on top (page 24)
- Extend legs long in front of you, ankles crossed
- Grip the pole between your thighs
- Roll your thighs in towards each other all the time
- Walk hands down the pole
- Slowly lower your body as your legs lift to the ceiling
- Let the pole move to just above your knees and hang back
- You can flex underneath foot for extra lock and hold
- To exit - return back up or Handstand

GSM's notes

"Aim to get the pole resting just above your knees and squeeze, a great conditioning move for your abdominals if you go up and down in the movement. If your coccyx bone protrudes slightly, you might find this painful - try the Goddess (page 49) instead."

Your notes:

_____
_____
_____
_____

Level Four
Extended Butterfly

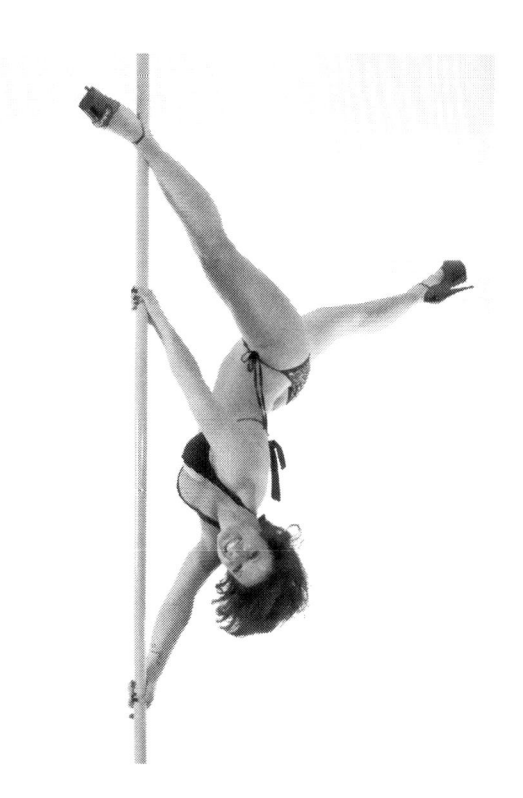

- Go into this just like the Butterfly (page 59)
- This time place your less dominant arm a little higher - so it pushes you slightly further away from the pole
- Pull up with the dominant arm and push with the less dominant arm
- Take your back leg off and extended behind you
- Let the pole slide down your leg on the pole to the back of the ankle
- To assist - keep your gaze upwards
- Keep body strong and lengthened throughout

GSM's notes

"If I place my bottom hand slightly higher up the pole, it pushes me away and up from the pole which is essential if I am to extend out in this move. The body needs to be pulled up, abdominals in. The trick is to nail the Butterfly first, then this move will come naturally as your strength increases."

Your notes:

_____
_____
_____
_____

Level Four
Pole Cat

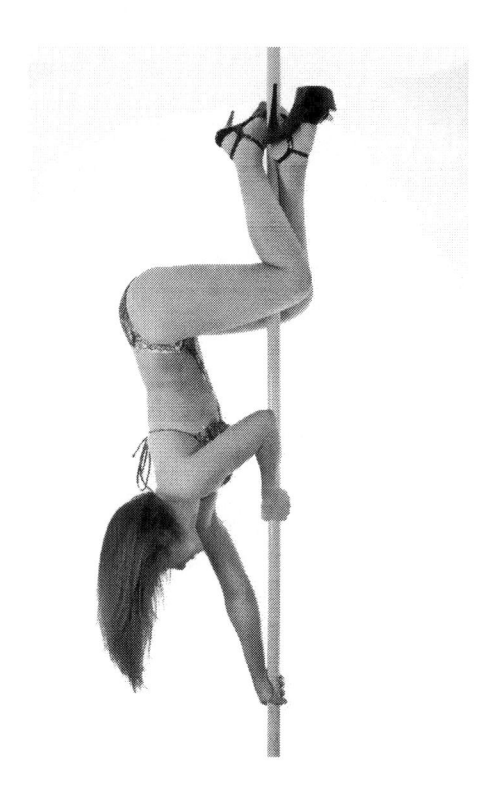

- Invert to Inverted Crucifix (page 51)
- Dominant arm to head height, less dominant arm to waist height
- Push arms and chest away from pole and grip between knees
- Here comes the hard bit - push your hips up against gravity, your less dominant arm will bend at the elbow
- Slide elegantly chest first towards the pole

GSM's notes

"Great strength move for you! Don't underestimate the amount of work involved pushing your body up against gravity. To keep secure on the pole make sure you have great grip between the lower legs around the pole."

Your notes:
_____
_____
_____
_____

Level Four
Half Bracket Invert Prep

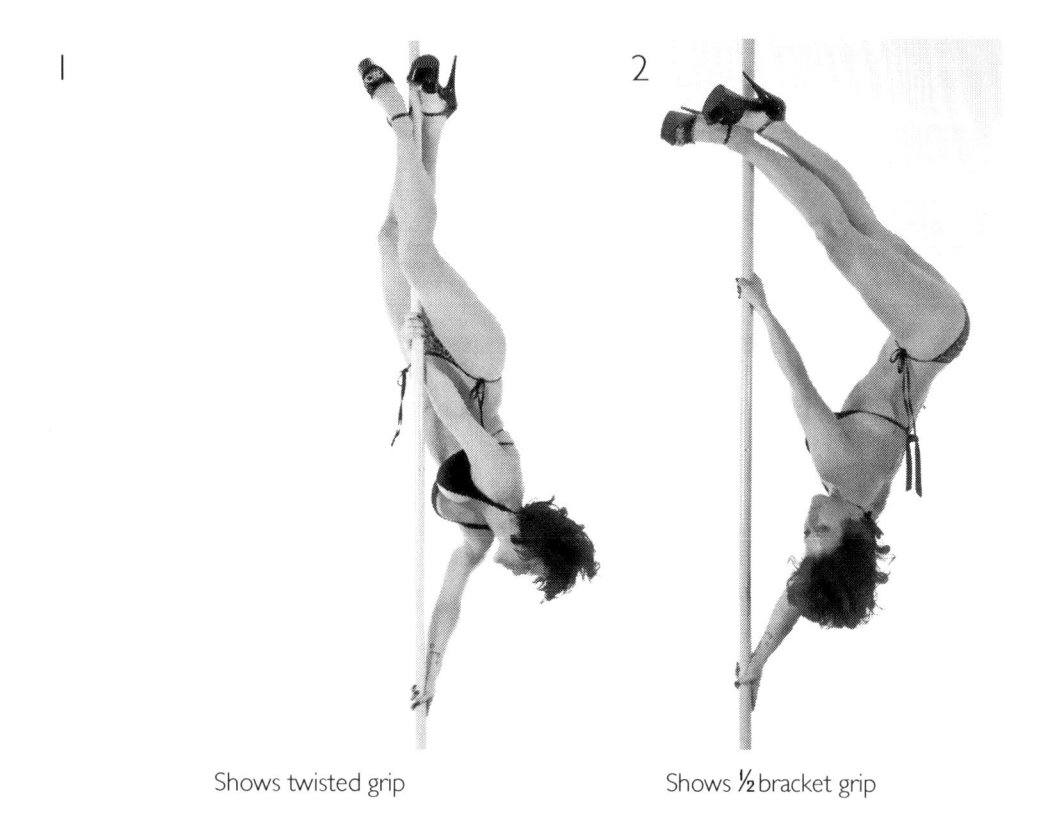

1

2

Shows twisted grip

Shows ½ bracket grip

- Note there are 2 grips to choose from twisted grip (picture 1) and ½ bracket (picture 2)
- Invert to Inverted Crucifix (page 51)
- Arms into ½ bracket grip or twisted grip (dominant arm is always on top)
- Pull up into the dominant arm and push with the less dominant arm
- Take the weight into the arms
- Lengthen through the spine
- As your legs slide down the pole your hips come away (picture 2)
- You are building up the strength in your arms and core so you can take the legs off in the full move (page 74)

GSM's notes

"You are really trying to move your hips and bottom away from the pole whilst keeping your body lifted up to the ceiling. Grip is essential for this move. Take your time practising this move."

Your notes:

_____
_____
_____
_____

Level Four
Full Half Bracket Invert

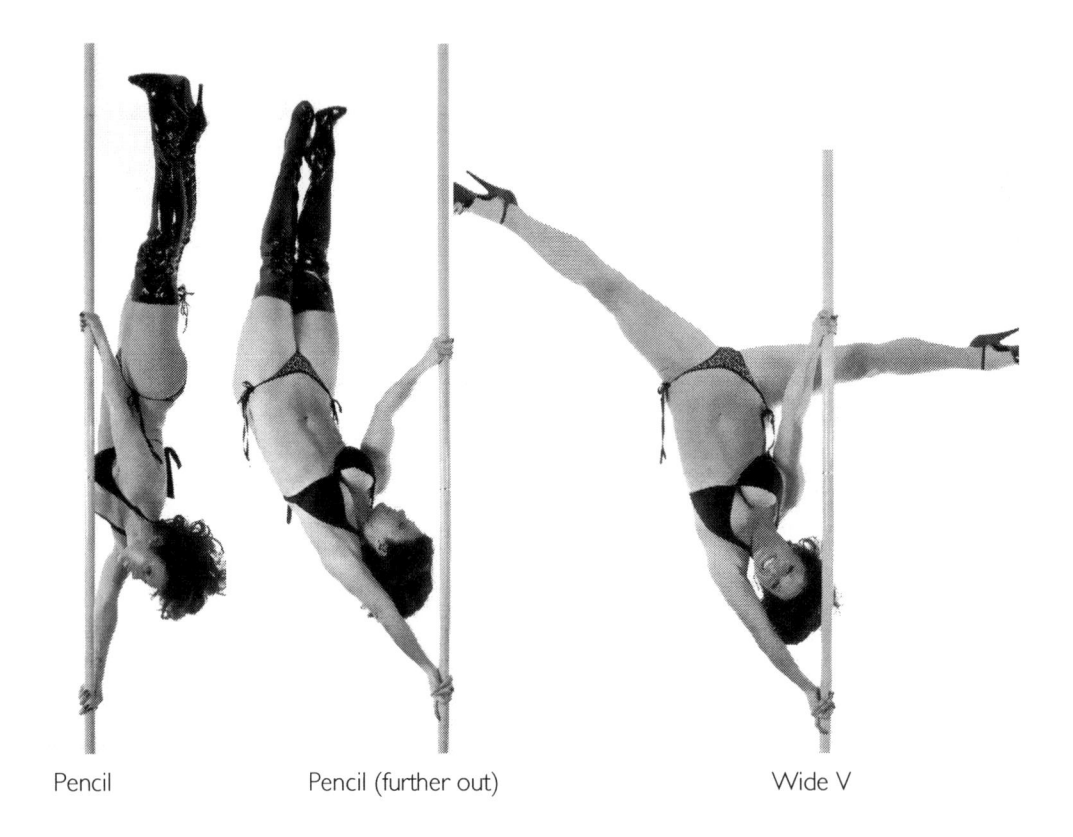

Pencil   Pencil (further out)   Wide V

- These positions will be yours with practice and dedication
- The wide V legs is the easier of the 3 positions
- Remember to pull up through your dominant arm and push with the less dominant arm
- Waist lines long

GSM's notes

"Please take your time with the prep for this move (page 73). As you start to feel more stable, you can start to take your legs off and move into the above positions. The wide V is the easiest to try first. Have a spotter on hand to help. All moves can be done 1/2 bracket grip or twisted grip. Please remember exiting out of this move is as important as getting in to it. Replace the legs back onto the pole with control. Also, with practice you will be able to lower yourself down to the floor with control."

Your notes:

_____
_____
_____
_____

Level Four
Super Invert from Shoulder Mount

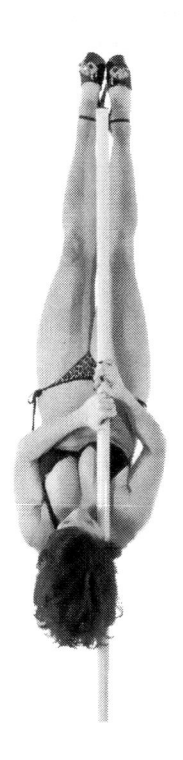

- Start with the Shoulder Mount (page 61) and go into a Straddle
- Extend both legs straight up to the ceiling and hold

GSM's notes

"It took me a while to get this, but as I gained more control and strength with my core this helped me to lift my hips higher. If you are coming back down out of this move make sure it is with control."

Your notes:

_____
_____
_____
_____

Level Four

Bow and Arrow

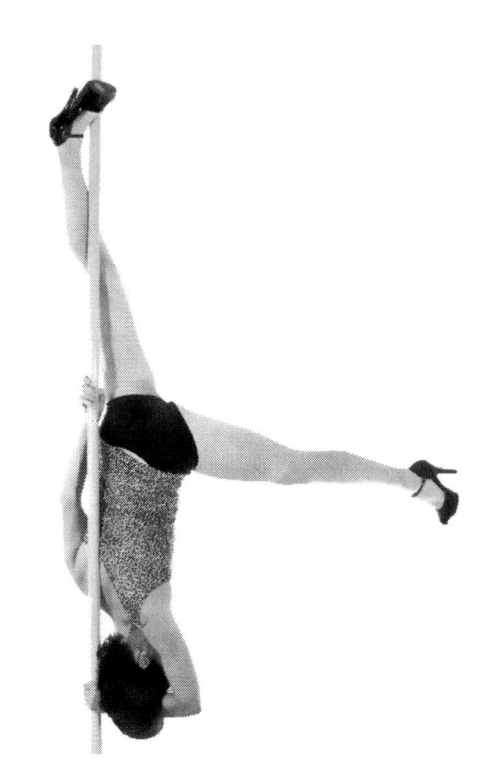

- From Straight Leg Release (page 70)
- Reposition hands - less dominant arm under head, dominant arm in to back
- Flex top foot to catch pole
- As other leg extends forwards over your body
- Reposition leg on to pole and slide out into a Handstand

GSM's notes

"Option - You can have both hands in your lower back (I prefer this). It's all in the grip with your hands. You can dismount by placing your foot on the floor or if you are feeling strong, return the leg back to the pole and pull back up to sitting. The more flexible your legs and spine are, the further away from the pole you will go."

Your notes:

_____
_____
_____
_____

Level Four

Straddle - no hands

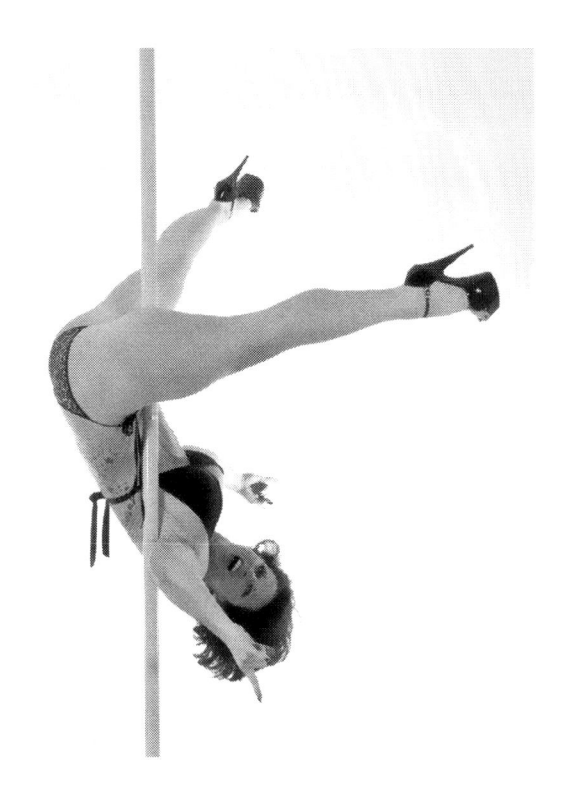

- Start in a Straddle (page 54)
- Pole sits in waist
- Take off less dominant arm and hold over the top of the inside thigh
- Squeeze into pole
- Take off both arms when you have your grip
- Optional rock hands!

GSM's notes

"The more I place the pole in my waist and armpit the more I am able to stick. Always when I am slightly warmer this move is so much easier."

Your notes:
_____
_____
_____
_____

Level Four

Reverse Shoulder Mount

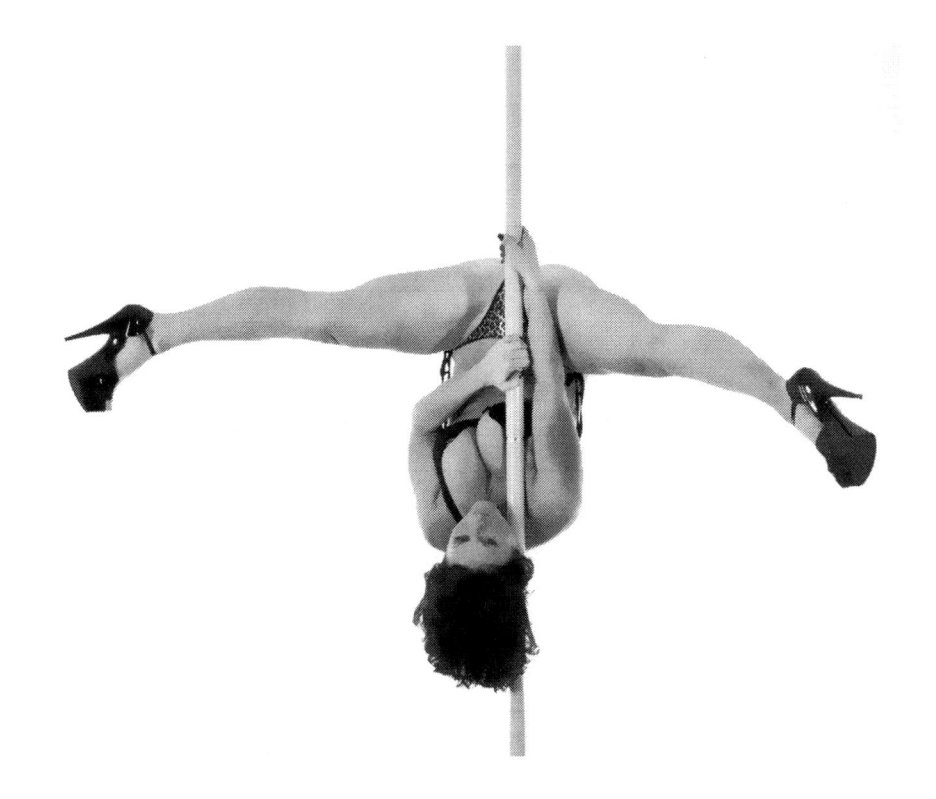

- The easiest way to co-ordinate yourself into this move is from a Shoulder Mount (page 61)
- Move into an Inverted Crucifix (page 51)
- Then Tuck yourself back underneath to Reverse Shoulder Mount out
- Note that I am using a different handgrip in this picture.

GSM's notes

"You can use a cupped handgrip for this one. For safety, it is best to lower your hips away from the pole first then control back down. Another sneaky strength move."

Your notes:

_____
_____
_____
_____

Level Four
Aysha Variations

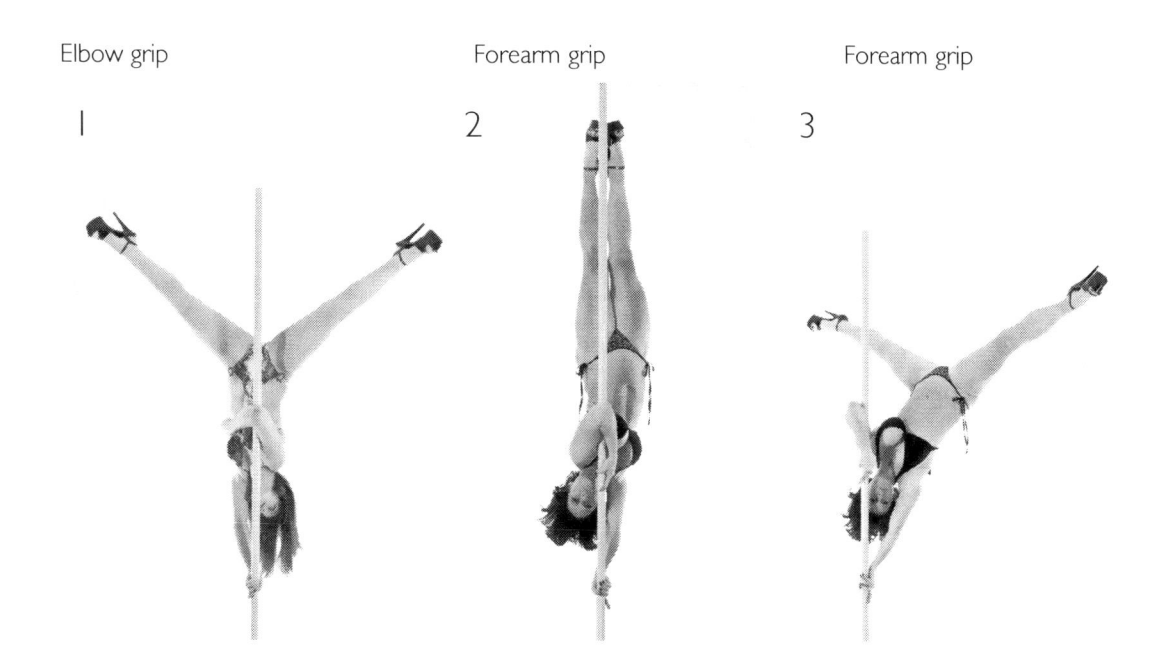

Elbow grip   Forearm grip   Forearm grip

1   2   3

- The Aysha has various arm positions: forearm grip (pictures 2 and 3) and elbow grip (picture 1)
- All the above moves started from an Inverted Crucifix (page 51)
- Elbow grip - dominant arm is underneath, less dominant arm is on top. Place the pole on the inside of the less dominant arm's elbow
- Forearm grip - dominant arm is underneath, less dominant arm is on top, hug pole in between bent arm and chest
- Always train to return to the pole with control

GSM's notes

"This baby took me sooooo long to grasp! Wobble, wobble but with perseverance I nailed this baby. Take your time and grab a spotter. The Aysha with the elbow grip works best when you are further away from the pole."

Your notes:

_____
_____
_____
_____

Level Four
Caterpillar Climb

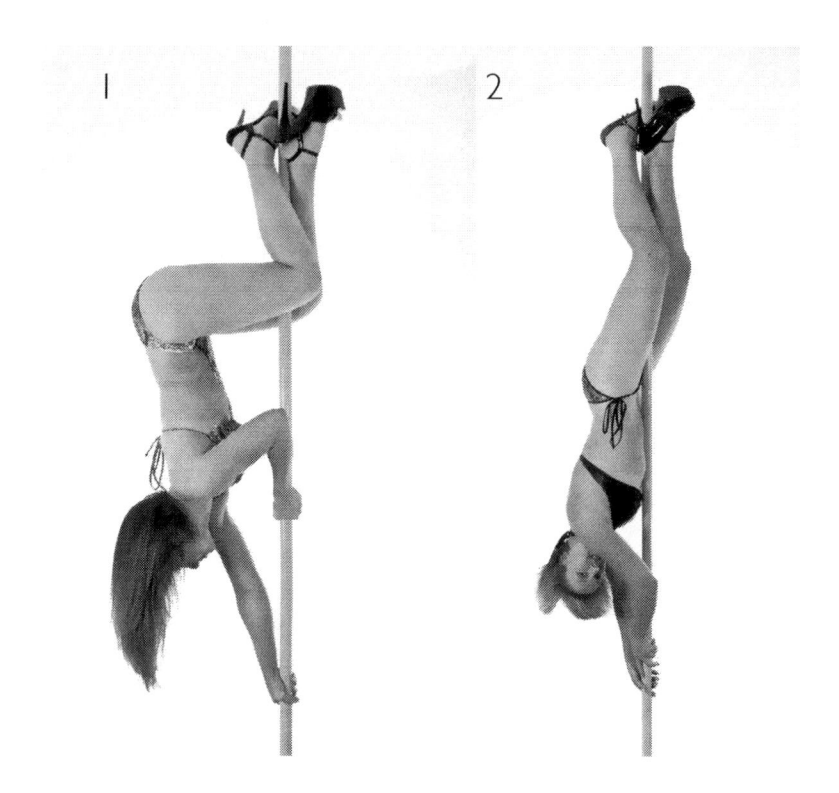

- Inverting to Inverted Crucifix (page 51)
- Then move yourself into the Pole Cat position (picture 1) with your hips high
- Have the pole in between your top arm and chest so you are hugging the pole (see picture 2 on page 79)
- Release the legs and replace higher up the pole (picture 2)
- Repeat

GSM's notes

"When I was learning this move, I was shaky and all over the place, in hindsight learning a great, stable Aysha will serve you so well. You will then have the stability to move up the pole. Practise this move with a spotter until you are really confident."

Your notes:

_____
_____
_____
_____

Level Four

Handspring

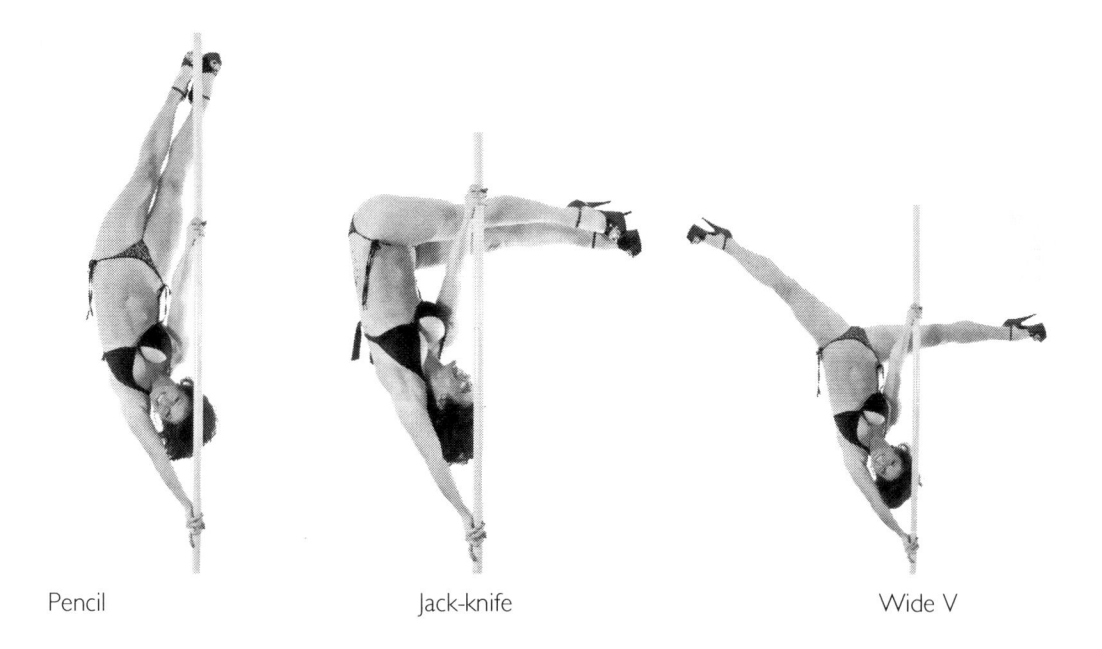

Pencil   Jack-knife   Wide V

- Start standing side on to the pole with the dominant arm next to the pole
- Place dominant arm up high and less dominant arm is low down - both arms straight
- Make sure pole is lined up with shoulders and chest
- Take a step back making sure you are still side on to the pole
- Please start with Prances - keeping your body very stable, kick back and land in the same spot. Repeat this to gain control. Prances are awesome to build up core control
- Once you have gained control, kick up higher whilst dropping your head
- Aim is to shoot the legs to the ceiling to hold
- Once you can invert - practise holding the other positions too, to build strength
- Lower down with control

GSM's notes

"This will take practice and dedication. Please do the Prances and land in the same spot - although it may feel like you may never get this, trust me, it will happen when your body's ready."

Your notes:

_____
_____
_____
_____

Level Four
Side Climbing

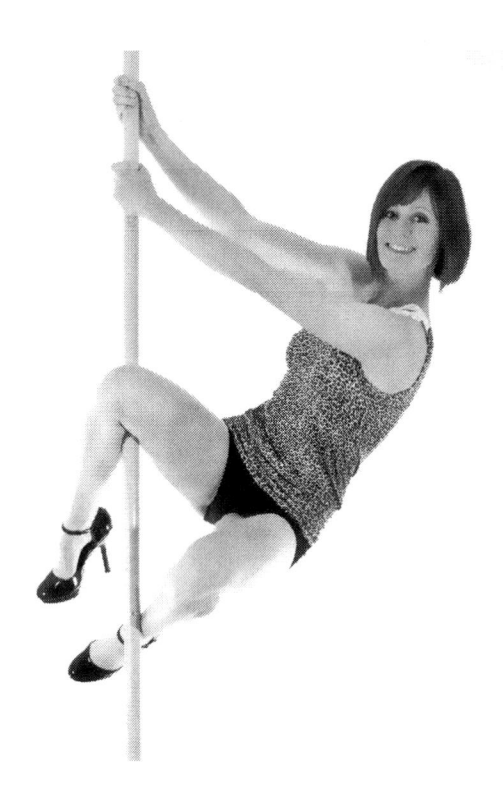

- Standing side on to the pole with your dominant side
- Less dominant arm low and dominant arm high
- Shoulders down and back
- Top leg hooked around the pole, bottom leg tucks behind the pole
- Using your arms, pull your hips closer to the pole
- Reposition your arm higher up the pole
- Then reposition your legs higher in the same position as before
- Repeat

GSM's notes

"I don't think that this is the most attractive way to climb the pole BUT it is awesome for increasing your strength and it is easy to transition into other moves up the pole, such as the Princess (page 57)."

Your notes:

_____
_____
_____
_____

Level Four
Teddy Bear

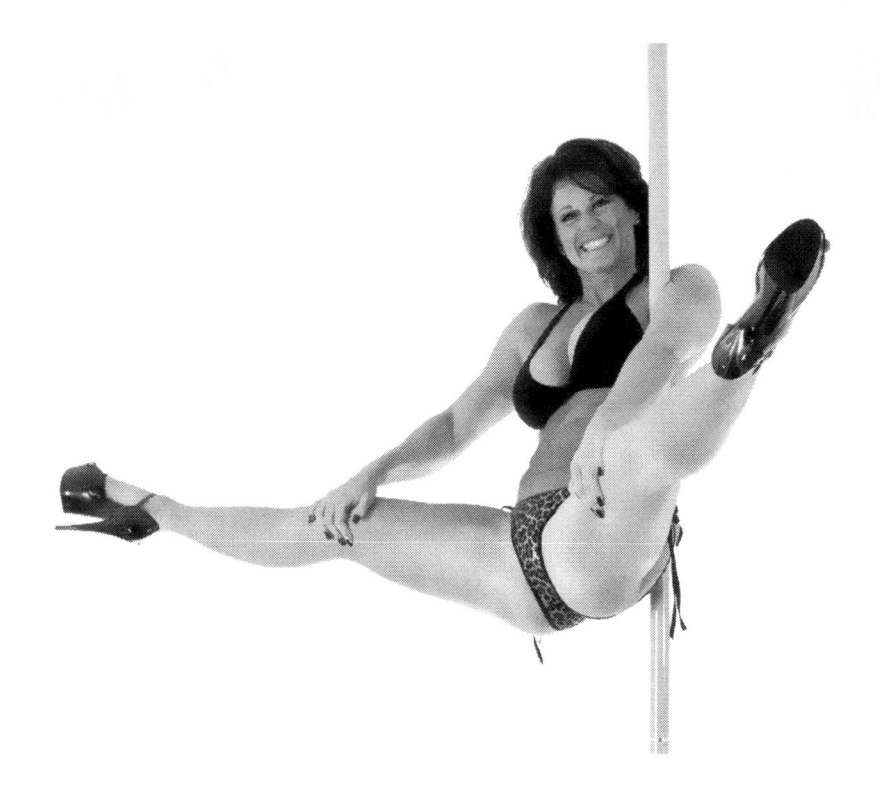

- Start from a Climb (page 25)
- Come forward of the pole on the same side as you would invert
- Less dominant arm is low and dominant arm is high
- Make sure your bottom is in front of the pole
- Take your less dominant arm off first and hold your thigh
- Test the waters to see if you are stuck to the pole by carefully removing your dominant arm
- If so remove the dominant arm and voila!

GSM's notes

"This one hurts, I can never do this if I'm cold and the pole is cold. My skin needs to be slightly hot so I will stick to the pole. Ooo, it hurts your armpit too!"

Your notes:

_____
_____
_____
_____

Level Four

Brass Monkey

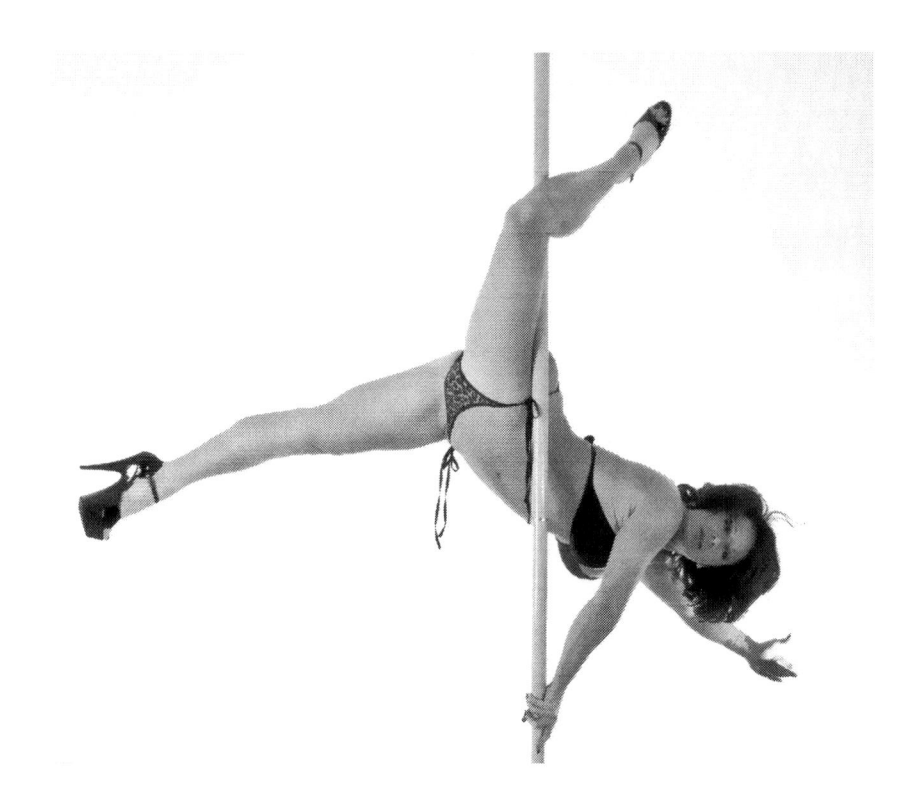

- There are numerous ways of moving into a Brass Monkey, I am doing this from a Super Invert (page 75)
- Once in your Super Invert, take both legs to the side of the pole where your dominant leg is closest to the pole. Hook your dominant leg onto the pole (mine here is my right)
- Grip with the back of your knee, point your foot and engage the muscles in your leg
- Take the outside leg forwards
- Then slide your hands down into a forearm grip or you can take one or both hands off

GSM's notes

"To enter this move you will need great core stability and control, it may take a while to get the control but don't rush. Also the more you engage your leg muscles the better your grip on the pole. To dismount you can hook your top foot onto the pole and pull yourself up or slide down to your hands. A spotter is essential when perfecting this move."

Your notes:

Level Four
One Handed Handstand Spin

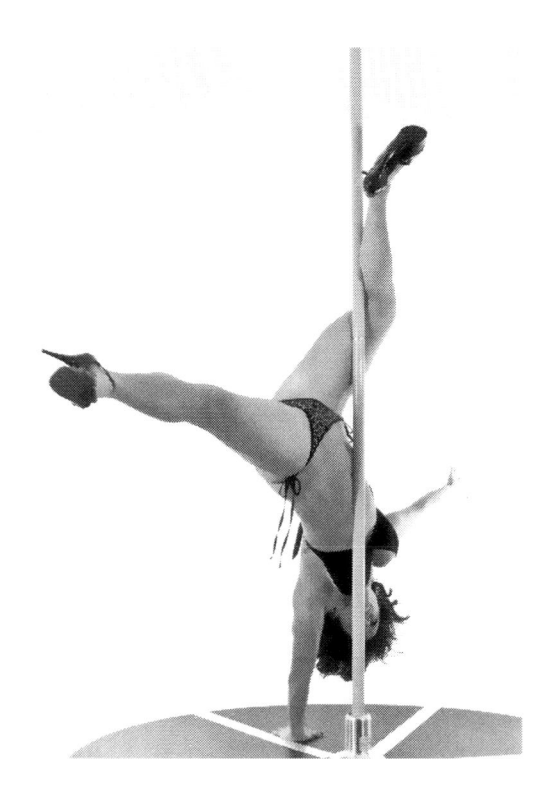

- From an Inverted Crucifix (page 51), slide down into a solid handstand (page 52)
- Weight is on one arm and legs go wide into a V
- Tip your weight over to your grounded arm and hook the pole into the opposite knee (back of)
- Sweep the other leg around towards the front of the pole and spin around into a Straddle (page 54)

GSM's notes

"You will need a solid, strong Handstand to do this. Also, most of my girls get a little scared of this move, as you need great balance too! So I suggest to them to practise with both hands on the floor to begin with."

Your notes:

_____
_____
_____
_____

Level Four

Flat Line Inside Hook

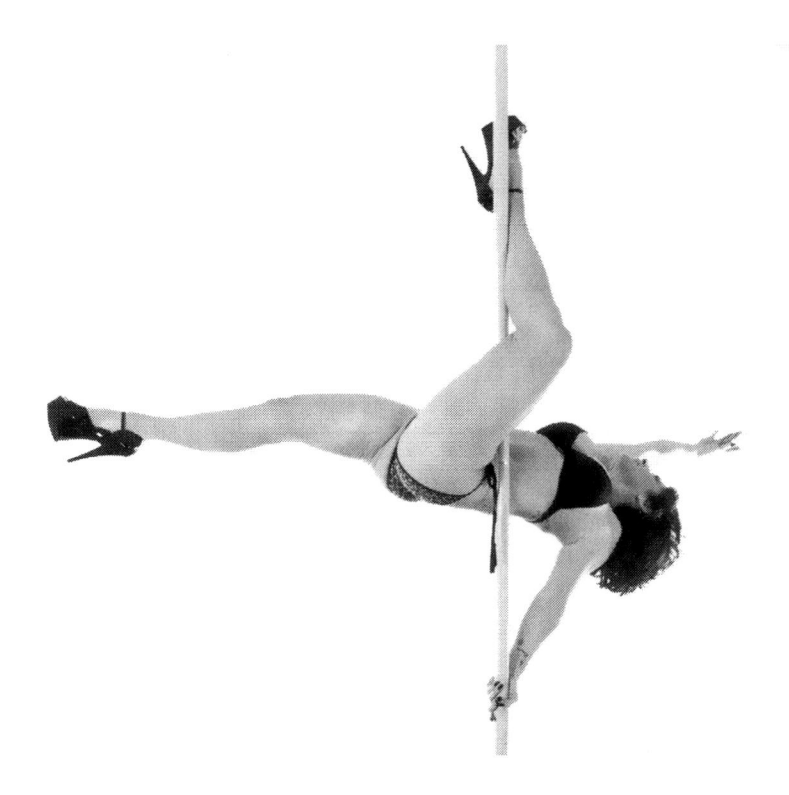

- From a no handed Inside Leg Hook (page 65) place the outside hand above the leg on the pole
- Bottom hand places underneath the body on the pole
- Extend outside leg straight out as you push up on the bottom arm
- Outside hand extends away

GSM's notes

"The more you hook your inside leg onto the pole the easier this move is to grasp. You can Straddle out to dismount or you can slide down the pole into the move on the next page..."

Your notes:

_____
_____
_____
_____

Level Four

Inside Leg Hook Handstand

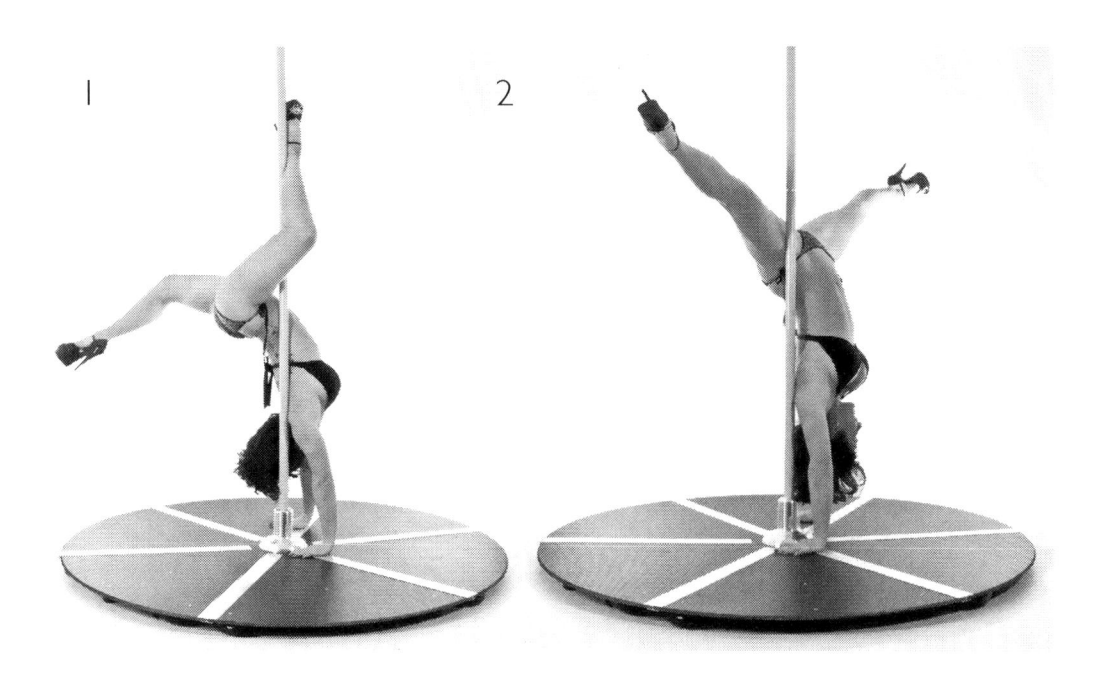

- From either an Inside Leg Hook (page 65) or a Flat Line Inside Hook (page 86), slide down to the floor into a grounded, stable Handstand
- Make sure the body is wrapped around the pole (picture 1)
- When stable you can open you legs out into a V (picture 2)
- To return up you can pull yourself up into a Flat Line Inside Leg Hook

GSM's notes

"Again the more you hook the inside leg around the pole the easier this move is to do as your body is naturally wrapped around the pole. You really need to stabilise your shoulders as well to help support your body weight."

Your notes:

Level Four

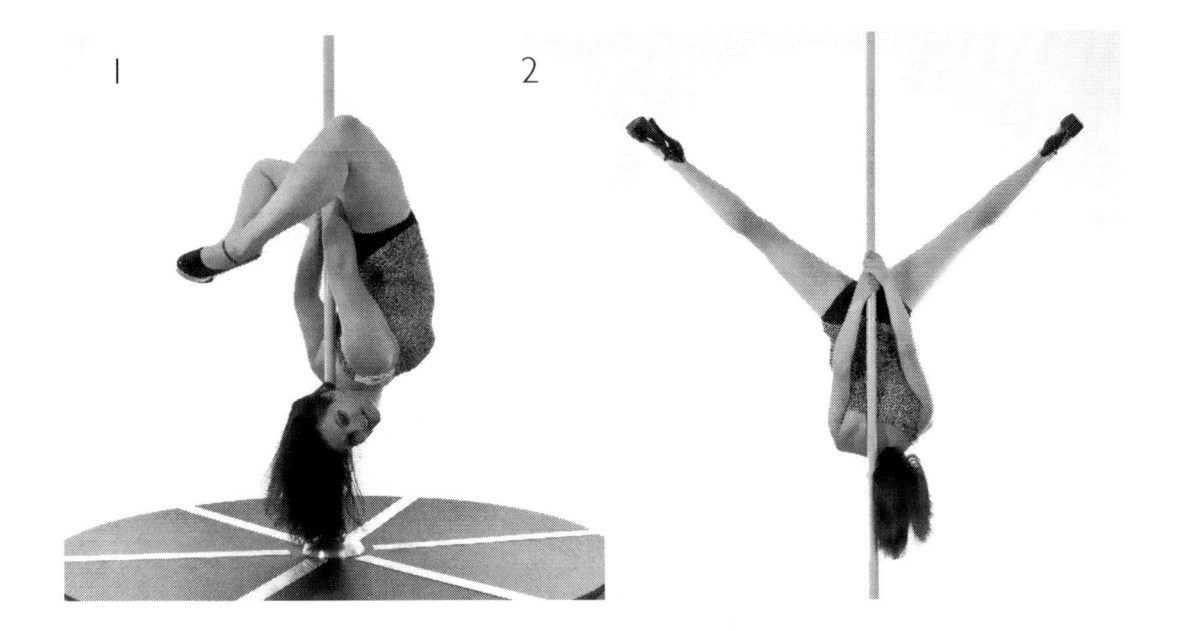

Jewel

- Face the pole and then bend forwards so your back is resting against the pole
- Reach arms up behind you and grip the pole
- Shoulders down and back and engage abdominals
- Lift your legs up slowly into a wide V - Sarah is demonstrating the Fang (picture 1) and Karen is demonstrating the wide V (picture 2)

GSM's notes

"When starting this move you may need a little momentum to get you up the pole and you can always hook your foot onto the pole to increase your confidence. You need great grip for this move too. You can also do this from a Straight Leg Release (page 70)."

Your notes:

_____
_____
_____
_____

Level Four

Knee Hold

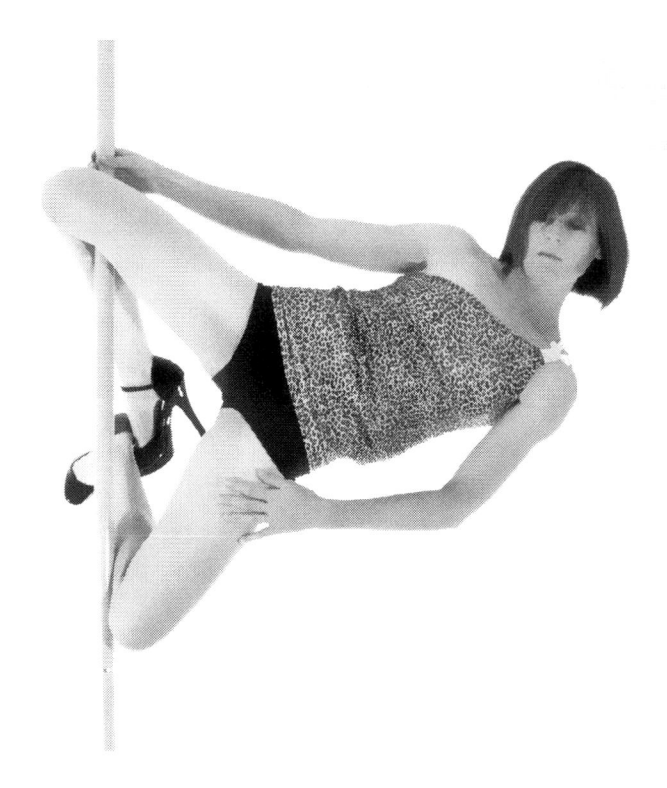

- The easiest place to practise this move is from the floor
- Hook the top leg around the pole with the knee higher than the hip
- Hands on the pole one above the leg and one below
- Place the other leg onto the pole with knee pointing down to the floor, pole rests just below knee cap
- Cross the bottom ankle in front of the top ankle
- Push your hips forward as you take away the bottom arm
- Keep yourself as horizontal as possible and when balanced remove top hand

GSM's notes

"The pain in your bottom knee area stops a lot of girls doing this move. The more you push your hips forward the easier it is to balance and hold. You really need to squeeze with your legs too to keep you on here."

Your notes:

_____
_____
_____
_____

Goddess Star Monroe's Expertise and Qualifications

Having spent over 20 years in the health and fitness industry, I have a wide range of qualifications and expertise. I am dedicated to learning and improving, being inspired and being inspiring. I seek out and find the most amazing people and teachers to grow and progress in my chosen fields. It's my pleasure to share with you my wide range of qualifications.

- Pole Dancing Community Approved School
- Level 3 - Advanced Instructor with the Register of Exercise Professionals no R0031775
- Post graduate diploma in Exercise and Health Behaviour - City University
- Sports Psychology Diploma
- Motivational Counselling Skills Certificate
- Lifestyle and Nutrition Style Facilitator

Pilates Training

- Stott Pilates Matwork Certificate
- M King Matwork Certificate
- Extensive training with PoleStars - studio and matwork
- Extensive training with Rebecca Leone - Pilates Excel Finishing School
- 2 year training with Pilates Foundation
- Studio and Rehab PATARA Gravity Reformer and Pilates matwork course

Massage Training

- Premier Sports Massage ITEC Anatomy, Physiology and Massage ITEC
- Aromatherapy
- Thai Massage Certificate Level I
- Thermo Auricular Therapist (Hopi Ear candles)

Fitness Training

- RSA Exercise to Music
- Chi-Ball Instructor
- Fit to Perform Personal Trainer
- Fit to Perform Health and Fitness Leader
- Fitness Professionals Pre / Post Natal
- Instructor Cardiac Rehabilitation
- Certified Fit to Perform Aqua Instructor

Yoga Training

- David Syes - Yogabeats
- David Swenson - Ashtanga Yoga Intro
- Jacqui Wan - Acroyoga
- Gabriella Roth - 5 Rhythms

Pole Dancing Training
- Caterina Gennaro
- Zoraya Judd
- Althea Austin
- Becca Butcher
- Maxine Betts
- Suzie Q
- Tracey Simmonds
- Jeyne Butterfly
- Felix Cane
- Tess Taylor
- Deb Riley
- Pantera
- Dana Myers
- Fawnia - Las Vegas
- Jada Fire - Las Vegas
- Shawn Frances Lee - Los Angeles
- S Factor - Los Angeles

Striptease and Burlesque Training
- Jo King London School of Striptease
- Immodesty Blaize
- Jeff Costa - Hollywood

Aerial Arts Training
- Studio Ohm - Las Vegas
- Aerial Showgirls - LA
- Circus Maniacs - Bristol Circus
- School - Turkey
- My Aerial Home - Beckenham

What other Pole Instructors say about Pole Dancing

Deb Riley

www.britishpoledanceacademy.com

My journey into Pole started the day I saw Panteras Pole Tricks 101 DVD, at the end of 2005. I just could NOT believe what I was seeing, "I want to do that", my heart screamed. I bought a pole and worked my way through the DVD. When I had got through it, I researched Pole teachers in the UK (there were very few around then) to try to find someone who was awesome at Pole Tricks. I couldn't, but it was a very different time then. There was literally NO pole dancing on the internet like there is today. So, it was extremely difficult for the pole dancers back in the day. This is why all the old-schoolers deserve so much credit. They paved the way and made it so much easier for the new generation to progress so fast.

My head went into overdrive trying to come up with exciting and dangerous poses. I was and still am absolutely fascinated with what I can get my body to do and am constantly pushing the limits of my strength.

After some time had passed I converted a room in my house into my first studio and began teaching. Fast-forward a further 5 years and with an unbelievable amount of hard work, I'm now the owner of one of the biggest pole dancing studios in the world - British Pole Dance Academy based in Stoke-On-Trent and I am considered one of the top instructors in the country. I'm also a Pole Tricks judge at Miss Pole Dance World finals and judge all the big competitions.

MY NAME IS DEB AND I'M A POLE TRICKS ADDICT!

Stacy Snedden

www.staceypole.com

I started poleing in January 2005, after taking my first class. I fell in love with it. Not being a gym bunny or into any other hobbies, pole just took over.

In September 2005, I became the Sales Manager of ' Vertical Leisure X-pole' - the largest pole manufacturer in the world. Once I started here, the clients I spoke to on a regular basis started to inspire me to instruct and develop my pole skills. As a larger lady, I went from a size 16 down to a 12 and became addicted! I found that both my work life and social life became revolved around pole dancing, making new life long friends along the way.

In 2008, I started my own pole school ' Stacey Pole'. After having a bout of post natal-depression with my first son Jacob, being able to pole and feel sexy, fit and great about my self again really helped me get over this and feel confident enough to marry my husband in 2010.

I have been VERY lucky to be able to travel the world with pole doing what I love the most and meeting some inspirational women (and some men) along the way.

I have now turned my hand to tour managing and currently manage tours for Justine McLucas, Alethea Austin, Karol Helms, Miss Suzie Q and Toby J, Amber Ray and Natasha Way.

Now with my personal dancing, after having my second child I am struggling to get back into pole. I am still touring and teaching but am now on a mission to get myself back into pole tricks. I will always love my dancing and still go crazy around the pole when a good song comes. I have always been proud of being a bigger pole dancer as I am proof that ANYONE can do this.

Sam Remmer

Joint founder of Pole Dance Community and proprietor of The Art of Dance

www.poledancecommunity.co.uk

www.theartofdance.co.uk

My journey into pole dancing started in 2004. A friend of mine had been working at the Windmill club in London and after she left she started to notice a negative change in her body shape and general fitness. We soon realised the fitness benefits of pole dancing.

As a novice, I was eager to learn as many pole-dancing tricks as I could. The Back Hook Spin was my first nemesis - it was taught to me by a lady from a local lap-dancing club and she performed the move so fast I could not interpret what she was doing but I was determined to achieve it and eventually I mastered it. The next stage was the Inverted Crucifix and the goalposts have continued to move ever since. I'm not sure if I will ever achieve the Rainbow Marchenko but will keep trying!

The rewards from pole dancing don't just come from my own personal achievements but also from watching my students' progression, I love seeing the students developing their fitness and self-confidence and I always come away from a class with a big smile on my face.

For me, pole dancing has become a lifestyle choice enabling me to keep fit whilst having fun. There is also a great social network that surrounds the pole-dancing world and I get paid for doing a job that I truly love.

Pippa Caesar

www.polenastics.co.uk

After months of trying to find the obligatory friend to go to a local pole dance lesson with, I finally discovered that one of my friends was already going! She assured me that it was NOT full of 19yr old Barbie dolls and that even though I was almost 36 and weighed around 13 stone, I was not going to be the oldest or largest in the class and didn't need to bring a bikini and get a full body wax.

That Thursday evening I was blown away. It was so incredibly hard and there were girls going upside down and all sorts. I LOVED it. I wanted to be able to do what those other girls in the class could do. I wanted to spin and climb and go upside down (the hardest move anyone knew at that time was an Inside Leg Hang!) so I signed up for the 6 weeks course and haven't looked back since.

Pole has changed my body shape, toned my physique, changed my personality for the better, it's made me stronger inside and out and made me so much more confident. I really enjoy getting fit and this is something I can have fun doing. I have met some amazing people, have collected some simply outstanding and supportive friends through attending pole classes, and can't believe how much my life has changed just by going to that one pole class back in 2007.

I love teaching pole, love being part of this amazing industry, love working with such talented people and am so happy that I took the plunge and went to that first class. I have never looked back.

Tracy Simmonds

www.thepolestudio.co.za
www.traceysimmonds.com
www.pfasa.co.za

It has been nearly seven years since I discovered my passion for pole dance.

I was a little lost and misguided in my early twenties. I had already quit dance school by then and opted to study nursing, so I could get a real job. It was during the time that I was studying to be a nurse when I realised that playing on the pole was actually my favourite thing to do. I spent hours training on the pole day and night, but the time flew by because I enjoyed every second of it. I had no idea why I was doing it or what I was working towards but by the time I had qualified as nurse, I had won Miss Pole Dance UK, I had trained as a fitness instructor and I had begun teaching other people to pole dance. Shortly after that, I took on pole dancing and teaching full time.

Since the beginning, my excitement and passion for learning new things about pole dance has never waivered. Each and every week I find a new challenge relating to pole dance. Whether it is for a new routine, a new move, a competition, devising new ways to instruct or trying to educate the people out there on what we do and why we love it so much. Pole dance is a challenge for the body and mind. Anyone willing to undertake that challenge will enjoy the rewards.

I now live and work in South Africa. I am proud to have opened The Pole Studio SA. I continue to travel internationally to host advanced pole workshops. I also work for the Pole Fitness Association of South Africa. We are actively promoting pole dance for fitness and as a reputable and enjoyable form of exercise for everyone.

Olivia Lawrence

www.athenafitness.co.uk

It was 5 years ago when a friend of mine asked me to try Pole Dancing with her. I have always been into fitness and at that point had worked in the fitness industry as a Personal Trainer and Sports Massage Therapist for 5 years with my company Athena Fitness so I thought I would go along with her and try out the new fitness craze.

I can remember being so nervous before my first pole dancing class, standing outside the door to the studio and saying to my friend "why are we here? This is going to be so embarrassing!" By the end of the class I was beaming, I'd had such a fantastic workout and a really fun exhilarating experience with some great people.

I continued to go to pole dancing classes for the next 3 years whilst at university studying for a degree in Sport and Exercise Science. During this time I noticed lots of positive changes in my body that I never saw from training in the gym, however, the biggest change I saw in myself was my increased confidence and self belief. When I graduated in 2009 I decided that instead of going on to be a P.E teacher I would teach Pole Fitness instead. In August 2009 I started Athena Pole Fitness,(yes me, the one who was nearly sick with nerves before participating in my first pole dancing lesson) a pole fitness school in Gravesend, Kent, for women over the age of 16 of all shapes and sizes. I wanted to create a supportive, safe, fun, all girls together environment, which with a little help from some amazing co-instructors we have achieved. I have seen many women in our classes change in many physical ways such as toning up, slimming down and becoming stronger and more flexible, we have also seen so many women grow emotionally and become more confident and happy in their own skin.

Pole Dancing is an amazing art in so many ways, it has totally changed my life and I have met some wonderful people and made some fantastic friends. I hope to be still working with Athena Pole Fitness for many many years to come.

Kay Penney

www.polepassion.com

www.misspoledance-uk.com

www.worldpoledance.com

www.r-polefitness.com

I first tried a pole at a friend's party. Imagining I was the star performer (in my head), I danced like no one was watching and found I was a natural - or so people kept telling me! I was free, my sensual side was revealed and I quickly identified the many benefits from these beautiful and artistic movements.

My mum, my inspiration, who sadly died due to the destruction of cancer, always told me that to make a difference in this world you need to think out of the box, break a few rules and as long as you don't hurt anyone, go for it!! In 2000, I thought out of the box - I created Pole Passion. I found my solace in this sport and I identified a new form of fitness and dance. Luckily, with the support and non-judgement of my closest family and friends, I just had the guts to stand up and stand out as I always knew what the power of the pole had done for me and what fun I had had in the process. This, in turn has made me a much better person enabling me now to support thousands of others across the world, men and women, finding and growing my leadership qualities in supporting those around me.

Empowering is one of Pole Passion's key words. Our mission statement is "empowerment, confidence, fitness and FUN". I am living proof of this and every day of the week, one more lady has a breakthrough with their confidence issues. They use the pole as a metaphor for strength (something they can hold on to for support - mentally and physically). As I progressed through my pole career, another vision was created. I wanted pole dance and fitness to be available to all ladies (and men) so they could do those artistic, beautiful, acrobatic and gymnastic movements and techniques in public without the fear of being wrongly labelled as a stripper or a prostitute. So, I created the "Miss Pole Dance UK Competition" in 2005.

With the growth of our competitions worldwide "Miss Pole Dance UK" and "World Pole Sport and Fitness" (World Pole Dance), I believe now that pole dancing and fitness can now be viewed as a sport . By changing the words from "Pole Dance" to "Pole Fitness Techniques", it changes your perception right? It has all the components of fitness so yes, it can be viewed as a sport and over the years with hard work we now have accredited instructor training programmes written by me in my above quest to educate and make programmes available to all.

Caterina Gennaro

Poleates
www.poleates.net

Pole dancing has impacted my life in such a positive way. I feel better, sexier and more confident than at any other time. Not only does pole dancing benefit the body, but also the soul. This empowering sport has transformed me to become an all-round different person, all for the better!

My confidence has increased, I have built up strength and flexibility and I feel I am in the best shape of my life. My technique and training regime focuses on the movements and techniques that make for a more fluid, graceful, and athletic dancer. I believe the importance of transitions between pole moves is a basic fundamental for a balanced performance.

Pole dancing is the perfect sensual escape for me balancing my busy career and raising twins. With pole dancing, there are always new and fun tricks to learn so it never leaves me bored. Also, the dance itself is a tool for me to just to let my body move and not think about it. The art of pole dancing has become such an expressive and athletic form of exercise that benefits both the novice and the professional dancer. I really see such a change in my students, which I find so fulfilling.

I was very fortunate to compete many times in the finalist competitions and was placed first in the US nationals last year. I look forward to judging future pole competitions worldwide.

Pole Fitness has really changed my life in so many ways, most of all it has given me the opportunity to meet the most amazing people, and to both teach and learn from my fellow pole athletes.

Juicy Resources

Goddess Star Monroe
www.goddessstarmonroe.com

Mentor, muse and educator for women. I have a passion and unique skill for inspiring women to fall in love with being themselves. I'm on hand for advice, inspiration and education. Look out for my 2nd book "How To Be A Woman" - coming soon.

Where to buy a pole:
www.x-pole.co.uk

I have used X poles since they first came out. Easy to put up and take down, minimal care needed. Available in static and spin.

www.r-polefitness.com

Great freestanding poles.

Perfect pole dancing shorts:
www.shaktiactivewear.com

www.poleskiwies.com

www.sweetvixencouture.com

All sell great pole dancing shorts that cover up what needs to be covered and reveals what needs to be revealed.

Pole dancing shoes / boots
www.alternative-footwear.co.uk

When ordering your first pair of stripper heels you don't have to go too high - try the 5" platforms out first, as these are easier to walk in. Also, always check to make sure the base (where your foot sits) of your new stripper shoe is cloth rather than leather covered as this stops you slipping.

Liquid Chalk
www.megagrip.co.uk

A little goes a long way and can get kind of messy!

Dry hands
dryhandsuk@hotmail.co.uk
07432645424

A great product to help your grip.

Alcohol
Search for Isopropyl Alcohol (to clean your poles) on www.maplin.co.uk

Pole Dance Community   www.poledancecommunity.co.uk

Do you want to find a reputable pole dancing school near you? Then you need PDC - the best community that supports pole dancing schools and pole enthusiasts in the UK. They have a strict code of conduct for pole dancing schools.

Pole Magazine   www.pole2polemagazine.com

Pole Dance DVDs

There are so many pole-dancing DVDs on the market and I have bought most of them - here are three pole dancers that really stood out for me.

www.bobbispolestudio.com.au

I love anything produced by Bobbi, super sexy, super strong and super instruction. All instruction is performed on spinning poles.

www.jamilla.com.au/Shop.html

You can't go wrong with Jamillas comprehensive set of pole dancing DVDs. Awesome instruction.

Pole Motion featuring Justine McLucas

A great DVD showing you a ton of strengthening exercises great for improving your skills on the pole.

It goes deeper...

There is something much deeper that happens when you begin your pole-dancing journey. You start to become more in control of your body and your mind. You become stronger, more determined and focused and this cannot help but overspill into your life.

As a mentor and muse to women everywhere, I shout it from the rooftops that it is essential that as women, we are in control of our lives and our bodies so that we can in turn create the kind of life that we fully desire and deserve.

Big changes will happen - not only with your body, but also in your mind and therefore your life. Everything stems from our thoughts and when you begin to feel stronger and believe in yourself anything is possible.

A note from me to you...

Understand that you are unique and there is no-one else quite like you.
You will have your own wants and desires and your own dislikes and likes.
You are more than the colour of your lip-gloss and the style of your hair.
Understand that life is a journey not a destination.

Remember that you will fuck up and then fuck up again.
Know that you will fall in and out of love many times. Clock it up to experience.
Please trust that only you know what is best for you. TV, magazines, your family and friends do not.
Know that you are truly a wonderful, gorgeous woman who has so many talents.

Know that anything is possible if you believe so.
Know that the words you say to yourself again and again will either build you or destroy you.
Know that this life and body is your responsibility.
Know that you have to take chances, a leap of faith - just do it, go on I dare you.

Know the ultimate position of power comes when you finally accept who you are.
Please surround yourself with inspirational and happy friends.
You are not your family.
Read something inspirational daily.

Keep a journal.
Diets don't work - enjoy eating foods that nourish you from the inside out.
Move a lot, dance, cycle, run, skip, jump - just move.
Don't spend money you haven't got.

Stop and breathe.
Know that we all have imperfections - it's only the airbrushed models that don't.
Finding yourself is far more important than finding the one.
You are SO much more than a number on the bathroom scales.

Honour your own body's cycles and rhythms.
Whisper to yourself how fabulous you are, then shout it from the rooftops.
Accept compliments and give them out freely.
Know that the best love affair you can ever have is the one with yourself.

Wisdom comes from making mistakes.
People will piss you off, get angry, get over it and move on,
Don't worry about what people say about you. It's what you think of you that is important.
Be careful of the story you tell yourself - it's a self-fulfilling prophecy.

Look deep into your eyes and know that you are OK just as you are.
Be kind to everyone you meet, for everyone is going through their own shit.
Know that your thoughts are just thoughts and you can change them in an instant.
Walk tall and be proud of who you are.

Smile at yourself, at others - just smile.
Love is the greatest emotion, spread it everywhere you go.
Know that you will feel jealous and you will compare - that's ok but let it go - there is no one like you.
Honour that we are all part of something so much bigger than just ourselves.

And you need to know that you are utterly amazing inside and out.
The world is yours to do with what you want.

X

Remember I am always here to help.
www.Goddessstarmonroe.com
Star@Goddessstarmonroe.com

Printed in Great Britain
by Amazon